Your
Skin

Dr Graham Colver
Mark Evans
Penny Tripp

Published 1990 by
Harrap Publishing Group Ltd
Chelsea House
26 Market Square
Bromley
Kent BR1 1NA
By arrangement with Amanuensis Books Ltd

ISBN 0 245-60010-8

This book was designed and produced by
Amanuensis Books Ltd
12 Station Road
Didcot
Oxfordshire OX11 7LL
UK

Editorial and art director: Loraine Fergusson
Senior editor: Lynne Gregory
Authenticator: Dr Hugh Pelly
Illustration: Loraine Fergusson, Ron Freeborn, Lynne Gregory, David Gifford
Cover design: Roger King Graphic Studios

MGI Prime Health, the health division of Municipal General Insurance Ltd, part of the Municipal Insurance Group, has contributed to the cost of this publication.

The information contained in this book has been obtained from professional medical sources and every care has been taken to ensure that it is consistent with current medical practice. However, it is intended only as a guide to current medical practice and not as a substitute for the advice of your medical practitioner which must, on all occasions, be taken.

Contents

Your skin

Your skin is your body's largest organ. Depending on your size, it weighs up to about four and a half kilograms (ten pounds) and, if you could take it off and spread it out, it would cover an area of up to two square metres (two and a half square yards).

If you didn't have skin, there would be nothing between your delicate internal tissues and the potentially harmful bacteria and micro-organisms all around you. Those same tissues, and all your other vital organs, wouldn't be kept in the stable, temperature-controlled environment they need if they are to function efficiently. They would be at risk from your every contact with the outside world.

But your skin is more than just a passive barrier between you and your surroundings and a means of stopping your insides from falling out, though it fulfils both these functions.

Specialized structures in the skin are designed to receive and pass messages to your brain about what is going on around you. Others enable it to respond appropriately to that information. So your skin is sensitive to environmental changes, and can react to alterations in pressure or temperature that might otherwise harm it and the tissues it protects.

Unlike synthetic packaging, your skin can repair itself when it is damaged. As it ages, it renews itself. It automatically manufactures additional protection for particularly vulnerable areas, or those subject to especially heavy wear. Your skin grows as you do, and produces lubricating fluid to keep itself supple. It has the facility to make and store some of the substances essential for your body's health, and to help get rid of others that are not.

Your skin is thickest on the soles of your feet and the palms of your hands, thinnest on your eyelids. Whatever its thickness, your skin has two main layers: the epidermis (outermost layer) is, on average, only about 0.1 millimeter (1/250 of an inch) deep; the dermis beneath it is about four times thicker.

The epidermis

The epidermis is the part of the skin you can see, and

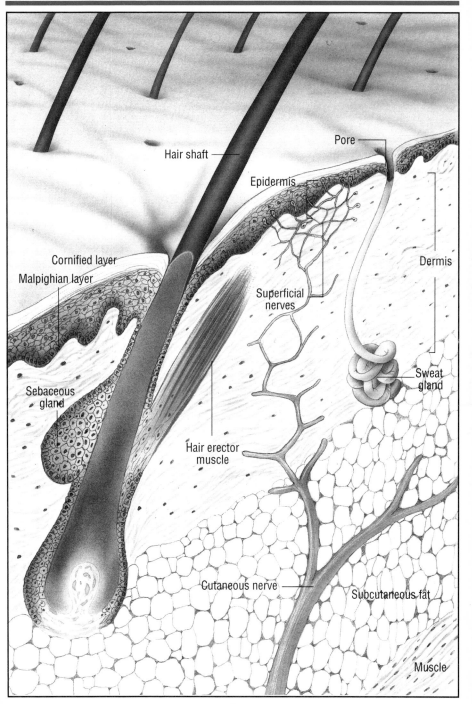

Hair shaft

Pore

Epidermis

Superficial nerves

Dermis

Cornified layer

Malpighian layer

Sweat gland

Sebaceous gland

Hair erector muscle

Cutaneous nerve

Subcutaneous fat

Muscle

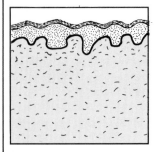

Skin color
The cornified layer is one way in which your skin protects itself and the underlying tissues against potentially-harmful environmental influences. Another is a brown pigment called melanin, made by specialized cells (melanocytes) in the Malpighian layer, and designed to protect your skin from damage by the ultra-violet radiation found in sunlight.

thickest on those areas of your body that experience the most friction - your palms, and the soles of your feet.

Wherever it is, your epidermis consists of three main layers of cells: the innermost Malpighian (germinative) layer, the granular layer, and the outer cornified layer.

How skin grows

Skin cells are constantly forming in the Malpighian layer of the epidermis, nourished by food and oxygen supplied from the dermis below. As they age, these irregularly-shaped 'prickle' or 'spiny' cells propel older ones towards the surface of your skin.

By the time they reach the granular layer, the prickle cells have become flattened and contain in their nuclei granules of a substance called keratohyalin. Chemicals known as enzymes work on the keratohyalin to transform it into keratin - a tough, fibrous protein.

On the thickest areas of your skin - your palms and soles - the cells pass through the granular stage to form an additional, clear, protective layer. Elsewhere they are transformed directly into the cornified (horny) layer.

Cornified skin cells are dead, flat and composed mainly of keratin. They are bound together into a strong, pliable membrane about twenty-five to thirty cell-layers thick whose primary function is to act as a defence against bacteria, heat, light and water. The cornified layer is continuously being worn away by friction, and replaced by younger cells coming up from beneath. Because this layer contains neither nerve endings nor blood vessels, you can damage it without causing pain or bleeding.

Around thirty days after it began to develop as a prickle cell in the Malpighian layer, the cell is shed from the surface of the skin. Some abnormal skin conditions mean that this process is dramatically speeded up so that in psoriasis, for example, cell production and shedding takes only about a quarter of the normal time.

Sunlight

Your body needs to absorb a certain amount of ultraviolet

light through your skin if it is to make vitamin D, essential for the proper processing of calcium in the body and the development of healthy bones and teeth. Only a tiny amount of the vitamin is available from foods.

Too much exposure to sunlight's ultraviolet rays, however, ages the skin prematurely, causes sunburn, and can increase your risk of skin cancer.

Dark skin has evolved as a way of protecting its wearers from the high levels of ultraviolet light found in the sunny areas of the world: in Northern Europe, however, where there is less need for such protection, fair skin means that people can absorb the beneficial amounts of ultraviolet light their bodies need.

When the pituitary gland in your brain detects the presence of ultraviolet radiation, it sends out a hormone which stimulates the melanocytes to produce increased amounts of melanin. Melanin has the effect of darkening your skin, so protecting its deeper layers from damage.

Whether you are a blond Northern European or a black African, you have around the same number of melanocytes in your skin. The difference is that dark-complexioned people produce more melanin, and it is found in all the layers of their epidermis. Fairer people only produce melanin in the lower epidermal layers.

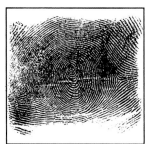

The papillary layer of the dermis takes the form of papillae (ridges) which interlock with the epidermis above it. The papillae are responsible for the unique skin patterns on your hands and fingers, and on the soles of your feet. Even after serious injury, your skin will grow back into the same patterns it had when you were born; only if the bottom layer of your epidermis is destroyed will the patterns change.

The dermis

Underneath the epidermis is the dermis, which gives your skin its resilience and pliability, and which is responsible for nourishing it. Like the epidermis, it is layered - the top (papillary) layer merges with the epidermis, while the undersurface of the lower (reticular) layer is attached to the subcutaneous (under-skin) layer of connective tissue and fat which insulates and protects the inner body structures.

The reticular layer is made up of a thick mesh of connective tissue, containing many fibers but relatively few cells. Its main component is a fibrous protein called collagen, also found in your tendons (muscle-to-bone connectors) and ligaments (bone-to-bone connectors).

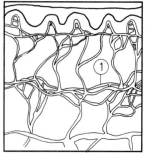

The rate at which blood flows through your skin is determined by your body temperature. The tiny arterioles carrying blood away from your heart are supplied with nerve fibers linking them with the heat-regulating center in the hypothalamus in your brain. When your body temperature is low the arterioles constrict (get smaller), the blood-flow through your skin is reduced, and you lose a minimal amount of heat through your skin. When your body temperature rises, the arterioles (1) dilate (enlarge), blood-flow through the skin is increased - and the excess heat from your internal organs is carried in your blood to be lost via the skin's surface.

Collagen is non-elastic and one of the strongest substances in your body: the collagen in the dermis gives your skin its strength.

Your skin's pliability comes from elastin, another fibrous protein in the connective tissue of the dermis. Elastin is also found in other parts of your body that have to stretch and change their shape and snap back, like your vocal cords, lungs and windpipe.

It is thought that both elastic and non-elastic fibers are made by cells called fibroblasts, which also play an important part in the skin's ability to recover from injury. The only other cells found in the dermis are macrophages, scavengers whose job it is to engulf and destroy invaders such as unwanted bacteria.

Blood capillaries

Each papilla of the dermis is supplied with a loop of capillaries. The blood in them carries nutrients and oxygen up to the Malpighian (germinative) layer of the epidermis, and to the various structures of the dermis itself, as well as playing an important part in the body's temperature-regulation system (see page 14).

The capillaries drain into veins, which join to form venous plexuses (intricate networks of veins) a few millimeters below the surface of the skin, and which contain large quantities of blood capable of heating the skin's surface.

Nerves

Your skin receives a great deal of information about its external environment through nerve endings in the dermis. The structure of the nerve endings varies according to the kind of sensation they are designed to receive: different kinds are sensitive to touch, pain, pressure and temperature.

Sensations from receptors in the skin travel along nerve fibers in the form of electrochemical impulses. Sometimes your brain is involved in your body's response to the messages received by the nerve endings in your skin; at other times, responses take the form of reflexes that bypass the brain altogether.

Though some nerves relay messages about sensations you are aware of, others are responsible for monitoring your skin's internal state. These collect information from structures like the blood vessels, sweat glands, and the muscles attached to hair follicles, and help to ensure that they perform their functions efficiently.

Special skin features

On or near the surface of your body are features associated with your skin which are closely related to its structure and functions, and are made from some of the same kinds of tissue, but which are not normally thought of as being 'skin'. These features include hair, sebaceous glands, sweat glands, and nails.

Hair

You have hair all over your skin except on your lips, the underside of your fingers, the upper side of your fingers from the top joint to the nail, and on the palms of your hands and soles of your feet. Each hair has a shaft that extends above the surface of your skin, and a root embedded in the hair follicle where it grows.

You even had hair before you were born. In the womb, babies are covered in fine down called lanugo. They usually lose the lanugo from their face and head about a month before birth, when it is replaced on the scalp by the longer, stiffer terminal hair. From that time, eighty-five per cent of the scalp is covered by terminal hairs, and the remainder by soft vellus. This vellus is the same fine, downy hair that covers most of your body for the rest of your life, sometimes so fine as to be almost invisible.

The distribution of body hair changes as you age. At puberty, when hormones stimulate your body towards sexual maturity, both boys and girls start to grow hair in their armpits and in the genital area. The influence of the sex hormones on hair growth is more noticeable in males than females, the most obvious sign being the development of hair follicles in the skin of the face to produce the coarse beard hair.

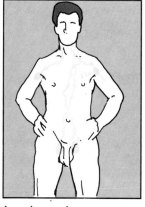

Lymph vessels
Though blood capillaries carry nutrients to the skin tissues they supply, the tissues are actually fed by a liquid called tissue fluid. This oozes out from the blood capillaries, bathes the tissues, and is then absorbed by vein-like structures called lymph vessels.

Lymph vessels run throughout the body, collecting up the 'used' tissue fluid (by now called lymph) and transporting it via the lymphatic system to the large veins in your neck. There it is returned to the bloodstream for recirculation as tissue fluid.

The dermis has a rich network of lymph vessels. They begin as lymph spaces at the tip of each papilla, and pass between the fibers of the connective tissue to form lymph capillaries in the subcutaneous tissue.

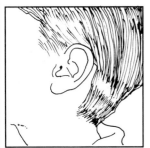

Terminal hair

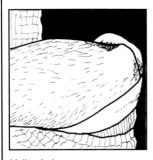

Vellus hair

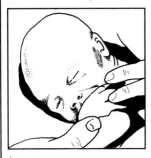

Lanugo

It has been estimated that you have about five million hair follicles in your skin: your scalp alone has around a hundred thousand of them. Some parts of your scalp are potentially hairier than others: on the crown you have about 300 follicles to the square centimeter, while on the back of your head there are about 200 in the same area. A man's beard has 30 to 40 hairs to the square centimeter, and you have around half that amount on the backs of your hands.

How your hair grows

The surface of the papilla is covered by a layer of epidermal cells, the germinal matrix. Hair is made when these cells multiply, and it grows as new cells are constantly added to its base. As the cells age, they change, becoming keratinized and dead like the skin of the epidermis.

By the time a hair emerges from the skin, it consists of a tough outer cuticle of thin, flattened, horny cells and a soft, fibrous inner cortex. In the center of the cortex is the medulla, made up of cells which lose their nuclei as they are pushed up away from the papilla, and containing the melanin which gives the hair its color.

The color of your hair is genetically determined, and depends on how much melanin is produced by your hair follicles. Melanin production tends to slow down as you get older, so that eventually new hairs may get no melanin at all and grow out white. No one knows why this should happen, but researchers have shown that white hair, rather than having melanin in its central shaft, instead has hundreds of microscopic air bubbles.

Whether you have straight or curly hair depends on the shape of your hair follicles and the way the cells in the papilla grow. An even growth pattern produces straight hair, which is circular in cross-section; curly hair is elliptical and produced by an uneven growth pattern. If your hair is coarse, it is because the cuticle accounts for around 10 per cent of each hair's volume; fine, flyaway hair is made up of 40 per cent cuticle and 60 per cent cortex.

Head hair grows at a rate of between 12 and 15 centimeters (5 and 6 inches) a year, while the hair on other parts of your body grows more slowly. It does not grow all the time: on your scalp, new cells are produced continuously for between two and six years before a three-month 'resting' period. At the end of this time, the hair root becomes detached from its follicle and eventually falls out. The follicle then rests for another three months before it again starts producing hair; around fifteen per cent of your hair follicles are 'resting' at any given time. Cutting hair has no effect on its growth rate.

Baldness

Alopecia, the medical name for baldness, seems in some way to be connected with male hormones called androgens. Androgens appear to be able to 'switch off' the center in a hair's root bulb that makes it generate new hair cells. Whatever the cause, the result is that scalp follicles stop making thick terminal hairs, and only produce vellus.

Baldness affects more men than women, and a certain amount of male hair loss with age is so common as to be normal. Typical 'male-pattern' baldness starts when hair begins to recede at the temples, then thin at the crown until a pronounced bald spot becomes visible. Balding continues at the back of the head until only a fringe of terminal hair is left. In some men the balding process slows down after the hairline has receded, in others when the crown has thinned out. Not all balding men end up with only a fringe of hair at the back of their head.

Women go bald, too, but their hair loss tends to be less noticeable than men's. Instead of falling out and leaving their scalp bare, women's hair tends to thin out everywhere, but not usually so much that the scalp is completely exposed. It is normal for women's hair to thin after the menopause, but severe stress and the after-effects of pregnancy and childbirth can cause dramatic (but temporary) baldness.

Temporary baldness or hair-thinning can also be a side-effect of certain illnesses, or the result of a diet that contains too few calories and too little protein. Illness or an inadequate diet may mean that the follicles are not able to produce hairs quickly enough to replace those that are lost,

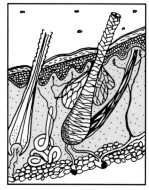

Hair follicles are deep infoldings of granular and germinative epidermal cells which penetrate down into the dermis. Hair growth only takes place at the base of the follicle, where it has expanded to form the hair bulb. The bulb is supplied with blood vessels, nerve endings and melanocytes (pigment-producing cells) by a small projection of dermal cells, the papilla.

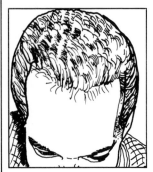

Male-pattern balding can begin as early as a man's early twenties and, because its cause is not yet fully understood, there is no known cure. Heredity does seem to have something to do with it, however: if a man's forebears were bald, the chances are that he will inherit the trait.

even though hairs are not being lost any more rapidly than they would be under normal circumstances. Temporary hair loss may also result when some illnesses are treated: chemotherapy used to combat cancer is one example.

What your hair is for

Body hair, wherever it grows, serves a useful function. Areas well supplied with thick terminal hair tend to be those at greatest risk from damage of one kind or another. The hair helps to cushion or insulate vulnerable tissues or organs, so protecting them from harm.

Body hair also acts like sensitive antennae, registering the slightest touch on your skin so that you are aware of potential danger. Pleasurable sensations, like those associated with love-making, are heightened by the increased sensitivity to touch of hairy skin.

Tiny hairs in your ears and nostrils intercept and filter out dust particles that would otherwise reach and harm delicate internal membranes. Your eyelashes, and the blinking reflex stimulated when they are touched, help keep foreign bodies out of your eyes; eyebrows act like miniature sweat bands to deflect perspiration.

Hair is waterproofed, lubricated and kept pliant by an oily substance produced from the sebaceous glands that open into each follicle. Also attached to the follicles are the erector pili muscles that run at an angle through your dermis, and over which you have no conscious control. Mammals that are covered in thicker hair than humans can use these muscles to fluff out their fur, increase the layer of trapped and warmed air next to their skin, and so reduce the amount of heat their bodies lose. It is a facility they also use when threatened, to make themselves look bigger and more frightening to a potential predator.

You still have the muscles that pull on your hair to make it stand up when you are cold or frightened, but the only consequence for your relatively hair-free skin is goose-pimples.

Sebaceous glands

Sebaceous glands are most numerous on your scalp,

forehead, cheeks and chin, but you have them all over your body apart from on the palms of your hands and the soles of your feet. The largest ones are on your face, neck and upper chest.

Although you are equipped with sebaceous glands from birth, their activity is low until the time you reach puberty. Production of sebum increases then as a result of the influence of sex hormones.

Sweat glands

The nail beds of your fingers and toes, and the edges of your lips, are the only places on your body where you do not have sweat glands. Like hair follicles and sebaceous glands, sweat glands are actually downgrowths of the epidermis, though they appear in the dermis. There are two kinds, eccrine and apocrine, responding to different stimuli and producing different kinds of sweat.

You have eccrine glands wherever you have skin, and these produce the greatest amount of sweat. They are especially numerous on the palms of your hands and the soles of your feet, and are also found in large concentrations on your forehead.

Eccrine glands are stimulated into action both by the temperature of your body's surface, and by your emotions. Sweating caused by stress occurs mainly on your palms and soles, and in your armpits.

Each eccrine gland has a glomerulus (secreting coil) buried deep in the dermis, and a duct to transport sweat from within the skin to the surface, where it emerges through a sweat pore. A network of blood capillaries surrounds the secreting coil, and the gland is also supplied with nerve fibers.

Sweating is one of the ways in which your body regulates its temperature (see page 16), but it is also a means of getting rid of waste products. Sweat from the eccrine glands is mostly water, but also contains sodium chloride (salt), urea (a by-product of protein metabolism also excreted in the urine), and lactic acid (one of the results of anerobic respiration, and toxic to cells). Traces of glucose, iron and ammonia are also present.

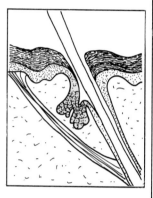

Sebaceous glands
Sebaceous glands are small sac-like structures made of epidermal cells. Most of them open into the sides of hair follicles (above) but some, like those found around the nipples and female sex organs, and on your eyelids, open directly onto the surface of your skin. Wherever they are, these glands produce sebum, a natural lubricant containing proteins, salts, cholesterol and fatty acids. This oil is important for lubricating your skin and hair, keeping them soft and flexible and protecting them from the effects of moisture loss and heat. Sebum also helps to stop the skin from becoming dry as a result of evaporation of moisture from within. The fatty acids in sebum are thought to play a part in preventing harmful micro-organisms and fungi from settling and multiplying on your skin.

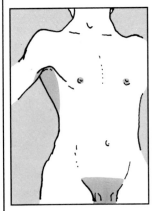

Apocrine glands are larger sweat glands, whose ducts open into hair follicles above the sebaceous glands. They are present at birth but only become active at puberty, and are found primarily around the genital area, in the armpits, and on the nipples and areolae. These glands produce a sticky, milky secretion which, like sweat from the eccrine glands, is odorless until it comes into contact with the skin bacteria that thrive on moist, warm surfaces.

Apocrine glands are stimulated by strong emotions ranging from fear and anger to sexual excitement.

On a hot day, or when you are undertaking strenuous exercise, you can lose up to 10 liters (2.2 gallons) of sweat in 24 hours, containing around thirty grams of sodium chloride. Cramp sets in if proper water and salt levels are not restored.

Nails

Your nails, like your hair, are modified forms of epidermal tissue stiffened by the protein keratin. They are tough enough to serve as a kind of armor-plating for the delicate tips of your fingers and toes, yet although they do not themselves contain any nerves, they are sensitive enough to pick up even tiny sensations when they come into contact with anything.

Blood capillaries in the nail bed give the nail plate its pink appearance, and supply the nutrients that keep it healthy.

It takes between three and six months for a nail to grow from the base of its nail bed to the tip. As it grows, it moves forward across the nail bed. Fingernails grow at a rate of about 4 centimeters (1.5 inches) a year, toe-nails at about half that.

Unlike your hair, your nails never stop growing, but they do grow faster at some times than others. Growth is quickest in your twenties and thirties, slowest in infancy and old age. Warm weather and pregnancy are associated with fast nail growth, but malnutrition and starvation slow it down dramatically.

The nails on your middle fingers and toes grow more quickly than any of the others, and it seems that the nail on the thumb of the hand you use most grows more quickly than the other one. It is not known why this should be so, but it has been suggested that the reason may lie either in the fact that your dominant hand is more active, or that more blood flows to it.

Temperature control

Human beings are warm-blooded animals, and can maintain a relatively constant body temperature even in extremes of arctic cold and tropical heat. This may be one reason why humans have a wider distribution across the world's surface than any other species: they are less dependent for survival on the temperature of their surroundings.

Environmental temperatures, both high and low, are not the only factors that influence your body temperature. Most of the chemical changes that take place in your body tissues during their normal functioning, in glands and muscles especially, generate heat energy. The heat your body tissues need is distributed to them by your circulatory system. If you had no way of getting rid of excess heat, your body temperature would rise by about 1°C every hour - even if you were not doing anything.

Constant body temperature is maintained by a balance between the heat produced and the heat lost by your body. When heat loss and gain do not balance, regulatory mechanisms in your body (which are under the control of the hypothalamus in your brain) come into action and compensate for overheating or overcooling. The temperature-regulating centers of your hypothalamus, one sensitive to heat, the other to cold, act like a thermostat, responding to information sent back from temperature receptors throughout your body.

Heat production

All your body tissues produce heat as a normal by-product of the chemical processes taking place within them. The greatest heat production is from the most active tissues - your liver, your glands and your muscles.

Muscular activity accounts for about thirty per cent of your body's heat production, even when you are resting. During physical exercise, the amount of heat your body produces is greatly increased.

Your body also gains heat when the environmental temperature is higher than your body temperature.

Heat loss

Your body loses heat through your skin by conduction, convection and radiation. Additionally, you get rid of a small amount in the air you breathe out, and in your urine and feces.

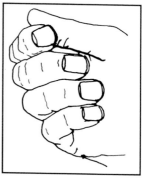

The part of the nail you can see is its clear body or plate, which is only 0.5 millimeter (2/10 inch) thick. It rests on a living, highly sensitive area called the nail bed, and grows out of the matrix (root) which is hidden under and protected by the cuticle at the base of the nail. It is the matrix that produces the new horny cells from which your nails are made, and the cuticle (the small flap of skin curving around the base of the nail) that guides the direction in which they grow. Also at the base of each nail is the opaque crescent-shaped lunula (half-moon), which is sometimes hidden under the cuticle.

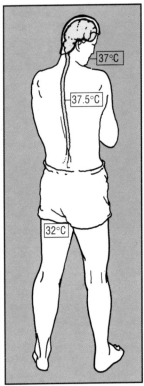

So that they can function properly, the temperature of your internal organs (the central, or core, temperature) must be kept at an almost constant level. The temperature of your skin, however, and the tissues just underneath it, can vary according to the environmental temperature - and needs to do so if your internal organs are to be protected and your vital systems safeguarded.

Radiation

Heat is transferred from your body's surface to objects nearby that are cooler; it is transferred to the skin by warmer objects.

Heat is carried from your internal organs to your skin by the bloodstream, and radiation of heat from your skin's surface can be increased greatly when the tiny blood vessels just under the surface of your skin get wider.

When the environmental temperature is higher than your body's temperature, you cannot lose heat by radiation.

Conduction

Heat is transferred from your body to any object or substance in direct contact with it. Rapid heat loss occurs when your body is in contact with good conductors of heat, like metal, or light cotton clothing, and can be minimized by wearing clothes made of wool or fur, which are poor conductors of heat.

Convection

Heat is transferred away from the body surface by the movement of the air around you. The air close to your skin is warmed by it and rises, allowing cooler air to take its place next to the skin.

Evaporation

Your body has to use heat to change water on the surface of your skin into water vapor. You continually lose a small amount of body heat this way by what is known as insensible perspiration, a process akin to sweating by which you get rid of about a cupful of water through your skin every twenty-four hours. You are unaware of insensible perspiration (hence its name) but it is a process that cannot be controlled for the purposes of temperature regulation.

When your body temperature rises, however, larger amounts of heat can be lost through sweating. The evaporation of sweat is a very efficient way of cooling your body, and is especially important when the environmental temperature rises to over 37°C (98.6°F) because under these conditions your body will gain heat by radiation, convection and conduction. In humid conditions, even if the air temperature is not especially high, sweat may drip off your body rather than evaporate on your skin, and therefore be useless as a coolant.

Preventing overheating

Overheating can result from a high environmental temperature, strenuous exercise, illness, over-exposure to the sun's radiation or a number of other external causes. If the temperature of the blood reaching your hypothalamus is a fraction of a degree higher than normal, nerve impulses are sent to your skin to cause vasodilation and sweating.

Vasodilation means that the arterioles (tiny arteries) under your epidermis dilate (get wider). As a result, more blood, carrying with it the heat from your internal organs, flows through the capillaries near the surface of your skin. In fair-skinned people, vasodilation may result in an obvious reddening of the skin on account of the increased volume of blood just below its surface. When the environmental temperature rises to 34°C (93.2°F), as much as 12 per cent of your blood may pass to your skin.

Sweating begins either when the external temperature rises above 29 to 31°C (around 86°F), its exact onset depending on the weight of clothing you have on, or when for any reason the blood reaching the hypothalamus is 0.5 to 1°C (1 to 2°F) higher than normal. Nerve impulses from the hypothalamus stimulate the sweat glands into activity. Fluid from the blood is filtered into the glands and passes through their ducts so that a layer of moisture appears on the surface of your skin. As the sweat evaporates on your skin, it takes the heat from your body and so reduces its temperature. It is evaporation from your forehead, upper lip, neck, chest and trunk that is responsible for temperature regulation: sweating from your palms, soles and armpits seems more closely related to stress than to raised body temperature.

In humid conditions, the air contains so much water vapor that your sweat may not evaporate quickly enough to produce adequate cooling. Heat stagnation, where body

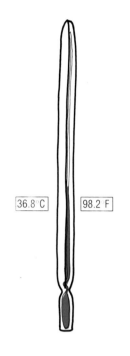

The average normal body temperature, the temperature of your blood, is 36.8 °C (98.2 °F) when measured in the closed mouth. Mouth temperature is considered to be the most reliable indicator of the blood temperature. 'Normal' body temperature varies - from one person to another, according to the time of day (it is lowest in the early morning, highest in the early evening), and depending on what you are doing. Readings of up to 1°C (2°F) above or below the average do not necessarily indicate ill-health.

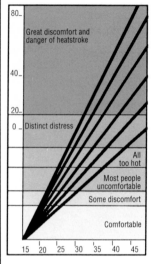

Heat stress
This diagram illustrates the way in which the temperature we feel is affected by humidity. The temperature is shown along the base of the diagram, the relative humidity by the diagonal lines, and comfort zones are defined by the horizontal lines. A high temperature is more tolerable if there is low humidity.

temperature rises to over 41°C (106°F), may be one result, and lead to collapse or even death. Heatstroke is another result of extreme overheating when, after prolonged sweating as a result of vigorous activity in high temperatures, sweat production ceases and the body temperature rises to a lethal level.

When a higher-than-normal body temperature is the result of illness, it is called pyrexia. This may be caused by toxins (poisons) from infecting organisms, or by protein-breakdown products from rapid tissue destruction. These substances act on your temperature-regulating centers, in time causing your body's thermostat to be reset at a higher level. As a result, your body is stimulated to go on to produce even more heat until its temperature reaches the abnormally-high level determined by the now-faulty thermostat. It is maintained at this level as long as the abnormal substance affecting your thermostat is present in your body.

Preventing overcooling

If your body begins to lose more heat than it is generating, your hypothalamus acts by cutting down sweat production and speeding up your metabolism (the rate at which chemical processes occur in your body) to increase the amount of heat your internal organs generate. The arterioles within your skin close up (vasoconstriction), so that there is a reduced loss of blood-heat through your skin's surface. Your muscles contract spasmodically in an involuntary reflex action (shivering) in order to produce additional heat. You get goose-pimples as the erector muscles attached to your hairs try to fluff out your non-existent fur in order to trap warm air next to your skin.

Sometimes, when heat loss is greater than heat production, your body cannot compensate quickly enough and the temperature deep within it begins to fall. This is known as hypothermia, and affects people - especially elderly, inactive ones or babies - who spend many hours in cold surroundings, or those who are exposed to cold, wet conditions for long periods. If affected by hypothermia, you become tired and weak, and eventually lose consciousness. It is a killer because your heart cannot function for long at abnormally low temperatures: if your body temperature is not carefully brought back to normal, heart failure can occur within a matter of hours.

Aging

Aging is not something that happens to you suddenly after a specific number of years has passed: it is a continuous process that affects both body and mind, the result of a combination of internal and external factors.

Skin aging is no exception. As you get older, the protein fibers (collagen and elastin) in your dermis change. They lose water as a result of a process called polymerization, and the result is that much of their flexibility goes. This is one reason for the skin wrinkles so characteristic of aging skin: another is that the subcutaneous (under-skin) layer of fatty tissue, which acts as a cushion for your delicate internal organs, loses some of its fat. As it disappears, the skin's supporting structure weakens. The skin itself begins to sag, and settles into folds and creases.

Another factor that contributes to the formation of wrinkles is an increased loss of moisture from your skin. Children have proportionately more water in their body tissues than adults do anyway, which is one reason why their skin tends to look firmer. Age slows down the activity of the sebaceous and sweat glands whose function is to supply the skin with moisturizing oils and water; elderly people's skin becomes increasingly dry as a consequence. The sebaceous glands slow down too, which also has an effect on your hair. It tends to become drier and more brittle.

With age, blood flow to the skin is reduced, the epidermis becomes thinner, and the blood capillaries near the skin's surface become more fragile. There is a decrease in the number of functioning melanocytes, the pigment-producing cells in the skin, leading to changes in skin color and the growth of 'white' (actually colorless) hair. Strangely, some melanocytes increase in size, producing

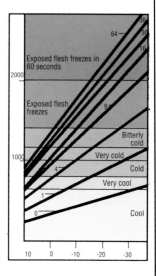

Wind chill
This diagram illustrates the cooling power of air on humans in different combinations of temperature and wind. The temperature is shown along the bottom of the diagram, and the units of windchill on the left hand side refer to kilogram calories per square meter of body surface per hour.

brown 'age spots' on the skin. All these changes happen anyway, but it is now known that the effects of the aging process can be accelerated by external conditions, like over-exposure to ultra-violet radiation. This puts the skin's delicate tissues, and its inbuilt protective systems, under more stress than they are designed to cope with.

Sunburn may have one short-term effect. Epidermal cells are damaged; blisters develop if deeper layers of the skin are affected. When large numbers of skin cells are destroyed, the production of new ones is speeded up. So many are made that they crowd one another to the surface, forcing the burned ones to peel off. Melanin production is speeded up, too, and it is the extra pigment produced by the melanocytes under stress that gives the skin its tan. The tan, therefore, is one of your skin's natural responses to injury by the sun rather than a symbol of a healthy, leisured lifestyle.

Although fair-skinned people are more obviously at risk from the harmful effects of ultra-violet rays (especially if, as many do, they expose themselves to fierce sunlight for a couple of holiday weeks a year) even those whose naturally darker skins are better able to protect themselves from damage still experience the drying (and aging) effects of prolonged exposure. Supplementing the skin's natural moisturizer - the sebum that coats the skin and hair, helping to keep it supple and forming a protective barrier to prevent excess moisture-loss from the body's tissues - with lotions or creams containing screening agents helps to minimize these problems.

You can slow down the effects of aging on your skin (by replacing lost moisture, or by exercise and massage which, by toning the skin's underlying muscles, help to maintain its firmness) but you cannot stop them. Neither can you unwrinkle skin which has begun to lose its resilience , except, in some cases, by surgery.

Plastic surgery

Plastic or reconstructive surgery first came to prominence after World War One, when many soldiers were badly disfigured by various kinds of explosive devices, but is now used routinely to help casualties of road accidents, those whose bodies have suffered mutilation as a result of surgical treatment for cancer, and burn victims (see Skin grafts, page 25).

Birth defects, webbed or extra fingers, cleft palates and genital abnormalities for example - can be corrected by plastic surgery, and it may be an option open to those who experience psychological suffering because they have physical features they perceive as being unacceptable or abnormal in some way. Some people see it as a way of dealing with the inevitable signs of getting older. Aging skin, which has lost its youthful resilience and become wrinkled, can be surgically 'lifted' so that it appears smooth.

Taking advantage of the fact that the collagen in the reticular layer of the dermis is arranged in bundles of fibers that form natural creases in the skin all over your body, surgeons can render scarring almost invisible by making their incisions along them. These creases, called Langer's lines after the scientist who first identified them, are of significance to plastic surgeons operating on any part of the body.

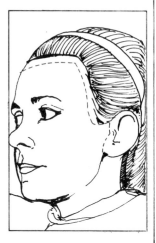

Creating a smoother, more youthful look for aging facial skin involves cutting into it on each side of the face - starting at the center of the hairline and running just in front of the ear - then continuing the incision round and behind the ear to the scalp. The facial skin is then separated from the subcutaneous tissue down to the chin. Unwanted fatty deposits are trimmed away and sagging muscles tightened before the surgeon pulls the skin upwards from the neck back over the face, and smooths it to fit over its new foundation. Excess skin is trimmed off, and the remaining flaps stitched back to the scalp. Healing takes only a few weeks but, because the actual aging process is irreversible and continues, the effects cannot be permanent.

Injury

Tanning is one of the ways in which your skin tries to protect itself from a specific form of injury. Another method it uses is to develop pads of thickened skin (calluses) as a response to long-term pressure or abrasion - on your hands or feet, for example. But because your skin is your body's first line of defence against invaders, it has other weapons, too. Nerve endings in your skin register information from the outside world, and warn you - via your nervous system - about potential dangers. If your body had no way of identifying and responding to pain you could, for example, be seriously burned before you realized you should move away from the source of the heat. Your skin contains different kinds of nerve endings (receptors) which register the different sensations associated with heat, cold, pain, touch and pressure.

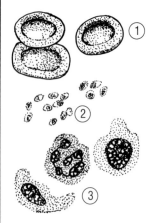

Blood consists of :
1. *Erythrocytes (red cells)*
2. *Platelets*
3. *Leucocytes (white cells)*
All are contained in a straw-colored liquid called plasma. There are around 5.5 million cells in a cubic millimeter of blood. It is the red cells which contain the pigment hemoglobin that gives the blood its colour, and which transport oxygen around your body.

Sometimes, however, your body's early-warning systems cannot prevent injury to the skin. When damage occurs, your body's own healing mechanisms - based on substances in your blood and the regenerative capacity of the skin's cells - are triggered, and can be supplemented when necessary by medical intervention.

Natural healing

Throughout the dermis all over your body runs a network of blood vessels carrying oxygen and nutrients to your tissues, and helping them get rid of waste products. These blood vessels may be damaged when your skin is injured, but even if an injury does not result in bleeding, your blood is involved in the healing process.

Leucocytes

To every 600 red cells, there is one white one. The actual number of white cells to a cubic millimeter of blood varies from 4000 to 13,000. There are three main types of white cell: granulocytes, lymphocytes and monocytes.

Granulocytes account for seventy per cent of the total of white cells. They are larger than red cells, irregular - and changeable - in shape, and they can move. They are made in the red marrow of short bones like the sternum (breast bone), ribs and vertebrae, and enter the circulatory system when they are mature by squeezing between the cells of the capillary walls. They live for about a week. Their job is to destroy bacteria and dead tissue cells by flowing around, engulfing and digesting them in a process called phagocytosis.

When your skin is injured or infected, granulocytes congregate at the site of the problem to devour invading bacteria and damaged tissue. The spread of infection is checked, and healing is speeded up.

Lymphocytes are smaller than the granulocytes, and make some of the chemicals called antibodies which combat foreign organisms in the blood. On average they survive for around one hundred days after being formed in the lymph nodes and spleen, but some are thought to live for years. About twenty-three per cent of the white blood cells are lymphocytes.

Monocytes, also made in the lymph nodes and spleen, can destroy almost any kind of foreign particle. They move into infected sites much more slowly than other white cells, so they are concerned with the healing of chronic (long-term) infection rather than acute injury.

Platelets

Along with the leucocytes in your blood, platelets (thrombocytes) play an important part in the healing process. There are between 200,000 and 500,000 of them in a cubic millimeter of blood.

Plasma

Plasma is the liquid part of your blood, and contains many compounds dissolved or suspended in water. It makes up about 60 per cent of your total blood volume if you are male, 64 per cent in females, and is about 90 per cent water. Some of its most important ingredients are the 70 or so plasma proteins which give blood its sticky feeling, and one of which, fibrinogen, plays a vital role in the healing of wounds.

When your skin is damaged - if you cut or scrape it, for example - the blood vessels in it are affected and platelets stick to the damaged area. The soluble threads of fibrinogen in the plasma are converted into insoluble fibrin, and a network of fibers is created across the wound. The fibers form a plug which stops any more blood leaking out of the damaged vessel, and prevents the entry of bacteria and poisons. This process is called blood clotting or coagulation.

The capillaries of the damaged area dilate (expand) and become more permeable, allowing plasma (along with its proteins) and leucocytes (white blood cells) to leak out into the surrounding tissues. This is what is happening when the skin around a wound reddens and swells.

Leucocytes combine with macrophages (stationary white scavenging cells) to fight any bacteria which may have entered the wound, helped by antibodies present in the plasma.

Eventually the dried blood clot shrinks, hardens and forms a scab which protects the damaged area while new tissue is growing. Underneath the scab, macrophages start to digest the blood clot and any cell debris. The fibroblasts (collagen-making cells) of the dermis speed up their production of new protein fibers to replace the damaged tissue. As the clot shrinks, the tissues it is protecting are pulled closer together, and the new cells made at the edges of the wound begin to spread over the inner surface of the scab. A new layer of skin grows at the rate of about 0.5 millimeter a day as the cells from the undamaged Malpighian (germinative) layer of the dermis multiply and migrate under the scab. As the regenerative process continues, new capillary branches develop from the damaged blood vessels. Damaged nerves regrow out into the tissues. Growth continues until the wound is closed by new tissue, and the protective scab falls off.

Scarring

An injury that affects only your epidermis will usually heal and disappear without a trace, but one that penetrates the outer layer of your skin into the dermis may sometimes leave a scar.

When your dermis is damaged, the fibroblasts making new collagen speed up their activity so that, instead of just supplying enough to ensure that normal growth processes can continue, they can replace destroyed tissue. If they create new fibrous tissue in large enough quantities, it is forced above the dermis and can be seen on the outer layer of the skin - a scar. Scar tissue is stronger and tougher than ordinary skin.

Though scars may first show themselves as slightly raised areas on the skin, they usually level off in time. Some, however, do not.

Known as keloids, these scars remain raised, shiny and smooth compared with the normal skin tissue that surrounds them. They often cover an area rather larger than the one originally affected by injury, and can develop after an operation or vaccination as well as following accidental injury. They occur because the fibroblasts do not shut down their extra collagen-producing facility when the initial wound has healed. Keloids are more common in black- or olive-skinned people, and their development is usually (though not always) associated with severe injury.

Burns

Burns can be caused by heat, chemicals or radiation, and vary in severity according to their depth. First-degree burns affect only the epidermis, causing pain, redness and some swelling. Second-degree burns affect both the epidermis and the dermis beneath, causing blistering, but the epidermis will usually regrow. Even partial-thickness burns like these can be dangerous if they affect a large enough area of skin.

Third-degree or full-thickness burns destroy both skin layers, and leave extensive scarring and dead skin.

Superficial burns which affect only the cornified or granular layers of the skin are usually repaired quickly by the new cells produced by the Malpighian (germinative) layer of the epidermis. Deeper burns which destroy the Malpighian layer heal more slowly, as a new germinative layer has to grow out from undamaged hair follicles to cover the exposed area. If the burns are so deep that the hair follicles are destroyed, scar tissue will still be produced by the dermis but a new epidermis cannot grow.

Extensive skin damage from burns or scalds spells danger for the body as a whole because of the skin's importance as a barrier against infection, and as a vital means of ensuring that your body maintains a stable internal environment. If large areas are lost, there is an increased chance of bacterial invasion and, as a result of the loss of plasma proteins and water, the onset of medically-defined shock.

Though partial-thickness burns normally heal themselves and mean no lasting damage to underlying tissues, full-thickness burns may require medical intervention in the form of skin grafting.

Skin grafts

If you suffer wounds that affect large areas of skin, or burns which have resulted in the destruction of hair follicles, they can be repaired by skin grafts. Small slices of skin, deep enough to contain the Malpighian layer and some dermis, are taken from a healthy part of your body and placed over the region to be covered.

After only a few days, the capillaries of the 'receiving' skin invade the 'donated' skin; within weeks, the graft becomes part of the damaged area. The skin of the 'donor' area heals normally as new skin grows from the remaining hair follicles; if a deeper layer is removed, healing is promoted by stitching the edges of the wound together.

Healthy skin for a graft has to be transplanted from your own body, as otherwise - unless you receive it from an identical twin - it will be rejected.

Researchers are tackling the problem of finding enough skin to cover a large wound in various ways - by cutting donor skin into fine strips which eventually grow together, by growing sheets of new skin from tiny fragments of donor skin in special nutrients, and by developing artificial skin from substances the body does not reject.

Acne

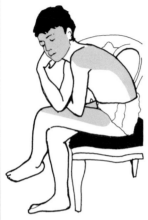

The spots of acne appear in skin where large sebaceous glands are found in association with hair follicles i.e. face, chest, shoulders and back. In severe cases the neck, buttocks, upper thighs and upper arms may also be involved.

Acne is something we all recognize. It is so common that only one person in three may escape and probably everyone has a little, mild acne at times. It is normal to have a degree of acne while growing up but this does not make it any easier to cope with. No one finds it easy to cope with any disfigurement on the face.

The first signs of acne are nearly always in adolescence. The peak for girls is between fourteen and seventeen years and for boys from sixteen to nineteen years. Once it has started there is usually a gradual deterioration for about four years, but in most people the acne disappears in the late teens or early twenties.

Different types of spots

Blackheads (comedones)

These are most common on the nose, ears and forehead and may be minute or easily visible. They consist of horn cells from the hair follicle, with melanin producing the colour. It is not clear why the horn cells stick together and fail to scale off the skin surface as they do in other body areas. But their retention in the opening of the hair follicle, as a plug, is not only unsightly but leads to other problems.

Increased greasiness (seborrhea)

Sebum is the name of the greasy liquid produced by the sebaceous glands. Acne sufferers nearly always have seborrhea. On the face there are about 600 sebaceous glands to a square centimeter and a small increase in their production of sebum soon leads to a greasy complexion.

At puberty, in response to rising hormone concentrations in the blood, the glands get bigger and more productive. The most important hormone is testosterone which, despite its more usual association with males, is in fact also found in females.

Papules, pustules and cysts

When sebum is dammed up in a plugged follicle it may leak out of the normal passageway into the dermis.

26

Bacteria may escape as well, and this combination seems to elicit the inflammation which is seen so often in acne.

The degree of inflammation depends on how much sebum leaked out, how many and which bacteria are present, how much squeezing and picking has been done and the response of each individual. Papules are small inflamed red spots which may last for a few days or a few weeks. Pustules have a yellow head and may develop from a papule. The pus discharges onto the skin after a few days.

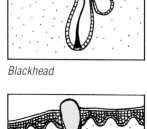

Blackhead

Cysts result from severe inflammation and often leave scars when they have settled; they are deep and push up the skin as though there was a marble buried underneath. The center is soft and the outside firm with scar tissue. They may be painful and sore to touch.

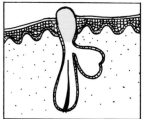

Scars

Some individuals are more prone to scarring than others. Generally the deep inflamed papules and cysts are more likely to scar but there is surprising variation between individuals. Scarring is of two types. One is lumpy and the other is due to loss of tissue giving a depressed area.

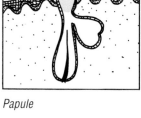

Papule

Hypertrophic scars are raised, smooth, pink lumps ranging from one millimeter to about one centimeter in size. They are most often seen on the upper trunk.

The second type of scarring may leave either a barely visible purple, flattened area which becomes white over a few years or a more obvious indentation. The hollow may either be shallow or deep and the deepest ones are less likely to improve with time. Generally the scars do get better eventually, and sometimes to a remarkable extent.

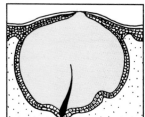

Cyst

Bacteria

There are plenty of bacteria on the skin and even more in the hair follicles. Many treatments for acne will also reduce the number of bacteria but that does not mean the bacteria are the main cause of acne.

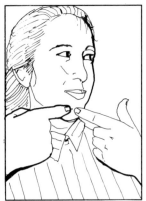

Picking
Most people pick at their spots a little and it usually slows the healing process rather than speeds it up. Some people, usually women, seem to be unable to leave their spots alone and decapitate every one with their finge nails: unfortunately such people are often quite obsessional and cannot break the habit.

Mild acne and avoidable acne

Acne usually starts as a few blackheads on the nose and forehead and a few inflamed papules also appear often on a greasy skin. Often the spots come in crops so that there are times in between without any spots. Many girls have a bout of acne around the time of their period.

Cosmetics

Very greasy or oily cosmetics are best avoided because they can block up the follicles and make acne worse. This may happen under a fringe when the hair may prevent the grease escaping. Disagreement about the best advice partly stems from the fact that in America they used to have a lot of trouble with greasy make-up causing acne. In Britain most doctors are happy to allow the use of non-comedogenic foundation, moisturizers etc. Some people gain much confidence if they can hide their spots.

Strangely it seems that some people who are obsessional face-washers, washing about six times a day, can also develop acne.

Clothing

Tight clothes and hot ones will tend to initiate acne spots. Headbands may cause acne on the forehead. Oil- or grease-soaked jeans or boiler suits may also cause acne.

Simple things you can do
Don't panic!

Many people regard the onset of a few acne spots as a disaster and they immediately foresee a spotty, scarred face staring back at them in the mirror. First it should be realized that most people's acne does not progress even to being moderately bad. Secondly there is very good treatment available for all grades of acne.

Soap and water will get rid of the grease from your skin and more expensive methods are not necessary. If your skin is sensitive it may be more comfortable to use unperfumed soaps. Do not wash more often than usual.

You should not let acne cramp your lifestyle but

some people find their spots are irritable when they are in hot, cramped, smoke-filled discotheques. People who play a lot of sport are often the types who can laugh off their acne and not let it get them down. Sunlight helps many people with acne: this is partly due to the camouflaging effect of a tan but there may also be a genuine reduction in the number of papules and blackheads. Simple anti-acne medication is equally effective, so artificial sunlight is rarely recommended as a treatment.

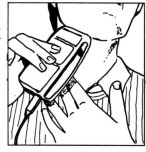

Shaving
If the spots are very sore it is best to avoid shaving. Less damage is done with an electric razor than with a wet shave.

Things which do not matter

For many years diet was blamed for acne. The notion that eating greasy food brought out the spots was common, and chocolate was considered the worst thing possible. Fortunately we now know chocolate to be innocent of this charge and in fact there is nothing to suggest that diet is involved.

Acne is definitely not infectious and should not interfere with physical contact with other people. It is not affected by too much or too little sexual activity.

Moderate and severe acne

It is difficult to understand why one person may have bad acne covering most of the back or chest but none on the face whilst another individual may have severe facial acne but little elsewhere. We presume that it is only the sebaceous glands and follicles in the affected areas that are responding to the hormone changes in the blood. Whichever area is affected, the changes are of larger papules and pustules which last longer and some of them may leave small scars. Blackheads will almost certainly be seen as well and they can be very extensive. When a flare-up occurs it may be very uncomfortable and an occasional cyst may appear.

Severe acne

Almost everyone will have known or at least seen someone with really nasty acne. They then expect their own acne

Coping with your acne

One of the most important reasons for reading a book like this is so that you can see your problem in perspective. First of all, although you may think that a few ugly spots on your cheek, appearing the morning before a party, is a disaster, that is not true. It would be a disaster to be involved in a serious accident. A few spots do not alter your appearance much. It is a matter of confidence; people frequently say 'Oh, he's alright - he's got enough confidence not to be bothered by a few spots'. You will know from experience that if you find somebody attractive then a few spots do not matter.

If people are mean and rude and call you names because of your spots you have to try to brush it off or ignore it. Sometimes it all gets too much and you feel miserable or depressed: you should then talk to your parents, another trusted adult, or your doctor. A lot of teenagers seem to think that their doctor will not be interested in their acne and the distress it causes. This is not true. Almost all doctors are happy to not only discuss the problem but to give advice about treatment.

will end up the same way but this is most unlikely. Roughly one in fifty acne sufferers has the severe form. It is often more extensive and the spots are deeper, more inflamed and last longer. Cysts may be quite a problem. Despite these changes the amount of scar formation can be minimal, but of course there are certainly people with pronounced scarring. It is for these people in particular that the most powerful modern drugs are reserved in order to treat the disease before more damage appears in the skin.

Treatment

Everyone would like a quick cure for acne but it is not possible. At first you may feel that you are not getting better but it is important to persevere with any treatment. One of the commonest reasons for failure of a medicine is stopping it too quickly: this applies to both skin preparations and those taken by mouth. Not every cream will suit everyone and some trial and error may be necessary. Most acne treatments come with instructions in the packing box and it is always worth reading them. They will tell you how often to apply it, how large an area of skin to cover, how long to keep going with it, whether you should soon go on to a higher strength and lastly, what sort of side effects to watch out for.

People with mild acne may not need any treatment at all but if they do it will always be a skin preparation. Those with moderate or severe disease can quite often manage with skin (topical) preparations alone, but failing this will need to take a medicine by mouth (oral treatment).

Mild acne
Over the counter
It is worth asking the pharmacist about the product you have seen advertised to check whether it really does have an active ingredient, which could help your acne, rather than ingredients which just make your skin feel better.

Killing bacteria
Bacteria are not the most important cause of acne but

there is usually some benefit from reducing their numbers. Agents such as hydroxyquinolone (found in Quinoderm cream and Valderma), chlorhexidine (Quinoderm face wash, Triać, Cepton), triclosan (Clearasil medicated, Oxyclean), will all do the job.

Blackhead removal
Removing blackheads is a useful approach, not only because they are ugly but because they also block the follicles and lead to some of the other changes of acne. Blackheads can be removed in three ways. First of all they can be removed by a blackhead extractor (comedone extractor) but these days such extractors are not used very much because the other methods are better. Clean finger nails should only be used if the blackhead is very nearly ready to drop out anyway.

The second method is by using abrasives which act rather like sand paper (see right-hand column). Another approach is the use of agents which soften the horny layer and this action helps to loosen blackheads. Salicylic acid is used for this, normally at a concentration of two per cent. Benzoyl peroxide not only loosens blackheads but helps to kill bacteria as well. It is the most widely used agent for this purpose and is found in preparations such as Oxy-10, Topex, Acnidazil, Ultra Clearasil, Acnegel, Panoxyl, Benzagel.

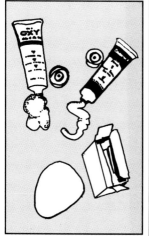

The lotion or gel contains millions of minute particles which are massaged over the blackheads. Various sizes of particles may be used and not everyone will suit your skin: the smaller particles are least irritating but least effective. Typical preparations are Brasivol and Ionax. Finally, there are pads available with an abrasive surface e.g. Buf-Puf.

Moderate and severe acne
Most people will need advice from their doctor to help in the treatment of moderate or severe acne. Generally doctors will start with cheap, safe agents which have few side effects and only if these fail will they recommend medication to be taken by mouth.

Topical preparations (onto the skin)
Benzoyl peroxide
This has been around for more than thirty years but we do not yet know fully how it works. It loosens blackheads and kills bacteria but has other effects as well. It comes in strengths from two-and-a-half to twenty per cent and

may be bought as a cream, gel or a wash. Examples are given in the previous section.

It is quite irritating to the skin for the first few days and may cause redness, dryness and scaling, but this varies between individuals. However, many people think that the redness it produces means that they are allergic to the preparation and so stop using it. Genuine allergy is very rare. If you persevere with treatment or perhaps stop for a few days and then start again, your skin will tolerate the benzoyl peroxide. It is best to start with a low strength and build up gradually. The full benefit of treatment is seen after several weeks and it can be continued for months or years.

Retinoic acid
Creams and gels containing this chemical are available and they help to loosen blackheads. They are not so good for inflamed acne spots. The chemical is marketed as Retin-A.

Topical antibiotics
Several antibiotics can now be applied to the skin directly e.g. erythromycin (Stiemycin), tetracycline (Topicycline) and clindamycin (Dalacin T). They penetrate the skin very well and kill bacteria in the follicles. Their main effect is in mild acne and some people find that after controlling more severe acne with other treatments they can keep it under control with a topical antibiotic. The lack of both staining and greasiness makes them popular lotions to use.

Oral therapy (taken by mouth)
Antibiotics
These are the mainstay of treatment for moderate or severe acne. Occasionally they may be required for people with minor acne who cannot tolerate topical preparations. Antibiotics kill bacteria but may have other effects as well. Only in the last few years have we reached a consensus on how much and for how long they should be taken. In the past they were often given in short

courses or in low dosage. Studies have now shown clearly that high doses should be given and for four to six months.

Tetracyclines are used most often and have very few side effects. They must be taken with water or an empty stomach, usually about half an hour before a meal. Minocycline is a special form which may kill bacteria more quickly.Erythromycin is another antibiotic acting in a similar way. Occasionally it causes an upset stomach.

Hormones

We know that androgens are important as a cause of acne and it is logical to try to counteract their effects. Two hormones, namely ethinyl oestradiol and cyproterone acetate are contained in a pill called Dianette. They both reduce the effect of androgens in different ways and provide a treatment for acne as effective as tetracycline. The treatment can only be given to females and has the added benefit of being an excellent contraceptive.

Retinoids

One member of this group of drugs is called isotretinoin and has been available for a few years to treat acne. It is a powerful agent which not only dries up the sebaceous glands, but helps to prevent the formation of blackheads. It is reserved for the treatment of patients who have failed to respond to antibiotics. The length of a course is usually four months.

It is an expensive drug and has several side effects including marked dryness of the lips and skin around the eyes and nose. It can also cause serious abnormalities in the developing fetus, so it is absolutely crucial that females have a negative pregnancy test before treatment and use proper contraception if they are sexually active. Only isotretinoin gives an improvement which is maintained for up to eighteen months after finishing the course.

Treating acne scars

If lumpy scars develop (hypertrophic scars) they can

sometimes be improved by the injection of a steroid preparation into the scar itself. Depressed scars are also difficult to treat but it is remarkable how much they improve with time. After the acne has settled the scars improve for up to five years. Very deep pit-like scars can sometimes be cut out: other treatments such as the injection of bovine collagen and dermabrasion are little used in the United Kingdom. Dermabrasion probably gives no better a result than natural healing but it speeds the process up.

Conclusions

Acne is very common and we now have good treatment for almost everyone, no matter how bad their problem. The treatment is always fairly lengthy and it is better if the individual follows instructions properly. Much can be done with simple remedies from the chemist but if this fails the doctor will have plenty of alternatives to help you. The psychological side of acne should not be forgotten because it can cause much distress but parents, doctors and your friends, will give you support and this, along with the treatment, will help you through your 'acne years'.

Birthmarks and pigment

Birthmarks

It would be logical if all birthmarks were present at birth. This is not always the case. Some marks appear in the first few days of life but others can be delayed by months or years. In these cases it is thought that the fault resides in the skin from birth but only reveals itself when some other factor acts as a trigger. An example of this is the unusual problem called Becker's nevus. It has the appearance, usually on the shoulder, of a large light brown patch, often with some coarse dark hair in it. It is first seen at puberty and is triggered by rising hormone levels.Salmon patches or stork bites derive their name from the old fable about babies being delivered down the chimney by a friendly stork whose beak has clasped the human bundle by the nape of the neck. These marks are seen in about a quarter of the population. Sometimes they are thought to have appeared in adult life but it is only that some new hair style or hair disease has revealed a patch that has really been present since birth.

The appearance of birthmarks in newborn children is deeply disturbing to the parents. There have always been individuals who see these marks as the sign of some maternal misconduct or in a biblical sense the sins of the father being visited on the child. This is not the medical viewpoint. We do know, however, that children born to alcoholic mothers, who have drunk heavily throughout pregnancy, are more likely to have birthmarks.

Stork-bite marks

Some birthmarks are caused by abnormalities in the blood vessels. If the capillaries (the smallest blood vessels of all) are wider than normal the skin will look red. Small red areas are very common on the back of the neck and, less often, on the forehead or upper eyelid. Fortunately those on the face usually disappear within a few months but on the back of the neck may remain throughout life.

Treatment is rarely required for these innocuous blemishes but if one persists in a visible area it is easy to cover with make-up.

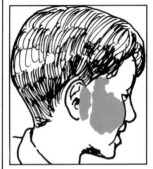

Port wine stain
Occasionally very wide capillaries are present from birth, causing an area of skin to appear flat but bright pink or purple. This is a port wine stain and in most people's minds is synonymous with a birthmark. It grows with the child and can be very disfiguring. With increasing age there is a tendency for the color to become more purple and for the surface to develop a velvety or even rough feel. Many port wine stains are in hidden areas e.g. upper thigh or chest and clearly these are not very distressing. On the face, however, they can have a great psychological impact on the person.

Port wine stains

Individuals vary greatly in how they cope with a port wine stain. Almost everyone goes through a stage of trying to hide it and many people do this successfully for a lifetime. Others eventually leave it uncovered. A range of camouflage creams is available and one can be obtained on NHS prescription (Covermark). Your own skin colour will determine which shade of cover to use. Thicker preparations may be required if the mark is not quite flat. Clinique have a range called Continuous Coverage, which are water-resistant, so that they will not run when you are swimming or exercising. The Clinique staff are well trained and are happy to put the creams on for you in the shop so that you can decide how well they suit you. This range is not on prescription and is quite costly. Excellent advice on all aspects of port wine stains and their treatment can be acquired from the Disfigurement Guidance Centre (see page 96).

The latest advance here has been with laser therapy and it is improving all the time. The problem with this form of treatment is getting the energy dose just right. Too low and nothing happens but too high can lead to scarring and it is more difficult to camouflage the stain if the surface has become lumpy. However, the tunable dye laser, which most people now use in preference to the argon laser, is unlikely to cause scarring and has the added advantage of being effective in the pinker stains of young children. These lasers are very expensive and treatment is not generally available. Within a few years it is likely that we will have them in a few major centres.

Strawberry marks

Another birthmark consisting of enlarged blood vessels is the strawberry mark. Although there was a vogue for removing them surgically whilst still large, most doctors now recommend no treatment. The exception to this is when a strawberry mark grows close to the eye and either obscures vision or pushes onto the eyeball. Treatment is then required to prevent permanent problems with sight. The other complication is bleeding from the surface: this can be dealt with by firm pressure over the birthmark with a dressing or clean handkerchief.

Moles

Some moles are present at birth but others appear later. The early ones are flat, brown marks with a well-defined but often irregular edge. Most are less than an inch in diameter but they can be much bigger. Very rarely one might cover much of the trunk or most of a limb. All these moles present from birth tend to be hairy. They grow with the child and do not disappear spontaneously.

The most common type of mole develops in childhood or less often in adult life. When examined under a microscope the mole shows an excessive number of melanocytes, the cells in the epidermis which produce pigment. Moles are so common that most people have between fifteen and twenty.

Most moles go through gradual changes. When we are children their commonest appearance is of a small flat, dark brown spot. During early adult life they have a tendency to become raised and for the shade of brown to change. They may stick out enough to get caught on clothes or jewelry. The surface may become warty or cauliflower-like. Eventually, when one has reached the mid-fifties most moles tend to get smaller again and to lose their color, so that in old age they are not a common sight. This description of the stages in the development of moles implies that a huge range of appearances may be compatible with a normal, harmless mole - e.g. they may be flat or raised, the shade can vary from skin-colored to black, the surface can be smooth or warty.

The range of normal moles has been stressed because people are becoming increasingly nervous about them. It is important to realize that most moles - even the odd-looking ones - are harmless. Having said that, it must not be forgotten that some moles can become cancerous, and that when a malignant melanoma starts to grow it can resemble a mole. There has been much publicity about this - telling people to keep a watchful eye on their moles. But please remember that this cancerous

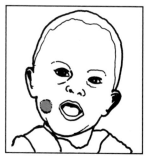

Strawberry mark

A strawberry mark is not usually present at birth but may appear at any time in the first few weeks of life. It then grows rapidly and may reach the size of a strawberry or even an apple.

Unfortunately this period of growth, which lasts a few months, is not followed by an equally rapid resolution. Instead it takes from four to eight years to shrink. Most strawberry marks disappear without trace or leave only a small blemish.

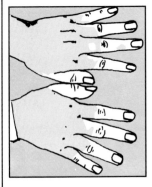

Vitiligo
About one in 200 people are affected by vitiligo and occasionally more than one person in a family is troubled by the disease. Pigment is lost from several skin areas, often on both sides, and the size of the white patches may increase for a few months. If improvement does occur it starts as small brown spots around the hair follicles. The pigment gradually spreads out and may coalesce to cover the whole area again. Unfortunately improvement is not the rule.

change only happens in about one person per 20,000 per year. What then are the important changes that suggest a mole is turning malignant? A rapid increase in size, obvious change in color and the edge becoming jagged are each sufficient to seek medical advice. Any of these may occur in a harmless mole but it is worth checking.

The doctor has to weigh up the odds when dealing with moles. If one is continually catching on clothing its removal may seem advisable. If there are obvious recent changes in a mole it may seem necessary to remove it to exclude an early cancer. Often doctors will be confident that there is nothing to worry about but if there is a nagging doubt they may take a photograph and recheck it a couple of months later to make sure there is no continuing growth or change.

Pigment

The pigment in our skin is called melanin and this same substance gives color to our hair and eyes. Fair-skinned people have only a little melanin while those with dark skins have a lot. The main function of melanin is to protect the skin from ultraviolet in the sun's rays. Most of the problems related to the skin and the sun are dealt with in another chapter but there are a few problems with pigmentation which are unrelated to the sun and they are discussed here.

Vitiligo

Intensive research, around the world, has so far failed to reveal the trigger for vitiligo or the mechanism. We know that antibodies against the melanocyte are found in the blood, that antibodies against the thyroid gland are also present but that they seem to do no harm.

The effect of vitiligo is mainly a psychological one. Fair-skinned people may not be troubled and some individuals notice it for the first time when they have been abroad and have acquired a suntan - only then does the white skin show up against the rest. In brown- or black-skinned races vitiligo is a far greater problem. The white patches stand out starkly, especially if the face is involved. In countries such as India it was confused with the effect of leprosy and could lead to a man being shunned by his people: in fact the two diseases are easy to distinguish and anyway no one has caught leprosy in Britain for over two hundred years.

Living with vitiligo can be made easier in several ways. A good sun-blocking cream is important to stop the white patches burning in the sun. Camouflaging the pale areas with Covermark, Clinique Continuous Coverage or other cream is especially useful on the face. There is some research into the use of PUVA treatment (as used for psoriasis) but it has not been fully evaluated yet. Useful information about vitiligo can be obtained from the Vitiligo Association (address page 96).

Chloasma
This is a darkening of the face, often giving a mask-like appearance. The forehead, cheeks and chin are most often involved. It sometimes occurs in pregnant women or those on the contraceptive pill and is therefore assumed to have something to do with the changing levels of hormones. It may last for months after delivery or stopping the pill but no treatment is known to help.

Pigmentation after inflammation
Many causes of inflammation can lead to melanin pigment escaping from the epidermis in the affected area. Examples are eczema, infection and burns. This leads to a darker color which may last for months - an effect more pronounced in people with dark skin. Care must be taken with proprietary preparations marketed for the removal of pigment because if the melanocyte is permanently damaged it may cease pigment production altogether. A cream called Fade Out is available and after several applications can produce a useful lightening of the color.

Lumps in the skin

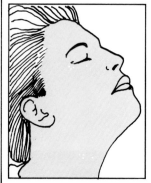

Milia
These are firm, white spots measuring up to two millimeters, and found on the face and neck. A frequent site is under or to the side of the eye and several may be present. They are small cysts of keratin but it is not clear why they form. No harm comes from them but they can be unsightly. Although they come and go to some extent by themselves it is possible to pierce them with a sterile needle and winkle out the contents. Another approach is to rub the surface with an abrasive preparation like Brasivol, the anti-acne preparation.

The medical meaning of the word tumor is simply a swelling or lump raised above the skin surface. Although some tumors are cancers, most are not and the word can be applied to something as harmless as a wart.

Harmless skin lumps of one type or another are exceedingly common: in fact everyone has one or more at some time in their life. Although moles, which are raised, could also be considered here they are dealt with in detail in the section on birthmarks and pigment. This section deals with both harmless or benign lumps as well as true cancers or malignant lumps.

Harmless lumps
Cysts
Sebaceous cysts sound as though they should be full of sebaceous fluid or sebum, but they are not. They are filled with keratin from a hair follicle or the epidermis. They grow most frequently on the scalp as firm rounded bumps and the size may vary from half a centimeter to that of a potato. Often more than one will develop and in some families there is a tendency to multiple cysts. The problem is usually cosmetic but a larger cyst may interfere at the hairdressers. If an infection develops within it, it becomes hot and tender and may discharge a nasty-smelling material. Unfortunately the occurrence of such an infection may interfere with its subsequent removal. In that case, instead of the sac being freed and pulled out through a small slit in the skin, it becomes stuck down, making removal difficult.

Skin tags
They are also known as fibro-epithelial polyps and are found mainly around the neck, in the armpits and groins. A typical specimen is a small, pear-shaped piece of skin. Often they are multiple and look like squashed mushrooms. The common complaint is that one or more catches on a necklace, shirt collar, vest, pants etc. Fat people have more skin tags than thin individuals and it is a good idea to lose weight if skin tags are becoming a

problem. The simplest treatment is to tie a piece of thread round the stalk and the tag will then drop off in its own time. They can also be snipped off with sharp scissors, and small tags will often not bleed.

Scars

Any significant injury will leave a scar which may be completely flat or raised. Some are bumpy, and if it becomes painful and bigger than the original wound or injury it is called a keloid. They may appear in acne scars, after surgery or after an accident. Some body sites are more prone to the production of keloids, the skin between the nipples and the nose, and the equivalent area on the back, being the worst of all. This is so to such an extent that doctors are much less keen to perform cosmetic operations in these areas for fear of a lumpy scar. Black-skinned people suffer particularly from this problem. While surgeons may be happy to deal with some types of ugly scar they will not want to do this in the case of a keloid because another and even bigger one is likely to occur round the new wound. Keloids can, however, often be helped by the injection of steroids into the scar.

Pyogenic granuloma

This is a less frequent response to injury, often seen in children and young adults. It is a red, round, often weeping tumor composed almost entirely of blood vessels. The site is usually where a pin, a thorn or some other sharp object has penetrated the skin. The finger, hands or lips are frequently involved. This tumor should always be seen by a doctor to check on its features and to arrange treatment. After the injection of some local anesthetic the pyogenic granuloma can be scooped out with a curette (sharp spoon-shaped instrument, see page 47).

Dermatofibroma

Yet another skin lump which in some cases is a response to injury. These are hard, brown or pinkish tumors measuring up to one centimeter across and they are rarely tender. The commonest sites are the skin and calves of

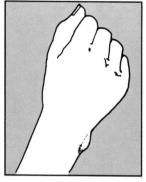

Ganglion
This swelling which contains a jelly-like fluid is found near a joint or tendon. The back of the wrist is a favorite place and it is common knowledge that in this site they were occasionally treated by being firmly hit with a large family bible. In fact ganglions usually cause little or no discomfort and in that case they are best left alone. If one is especially painful it can usually be removed by a surgeon.

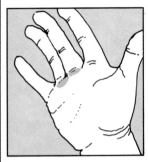

Corns and callosities are the responses of the skin to pressure. A callosity is a diffuse thickening of the outer layer (keratin) and it is a protective response to a widely applied, repeated friction or pressure. They are often related to work especially in manual workers but may also be seen for instance on the hands in tennis players and on the knees in floor-cleaners.

women. Dermatofibromas are completely harmless and in many cases are thought to be an odd scarring reaction to insect bites. Many will shrink over the years and it is not necessary to remove the lump unless it is unsightly or awkward, for example, lying beneath a shoe strap.

Corns and callosities
Callosities are nearly always painless and need no treatment. When the repeated friction stops the thickening slowly disappears. Corns and seed corns are seen mainly where there is a high local pressure and are commoner in the middle-aged and elderly. The typical site is on the foot where a bony area is pressed against a shoe, for example on top of the toes, and on the soles just below the base of the toes. On the soles they are often confused with verrucae but can be distinguished by paring down with a blade. A wart will be seen to have a rough surface, no normal markings and possibly black flecks of thrombosed capillaries. A corn, however, has normal skin markings and a solitary 'seed' of keratin at the center. Soft, soggy corns can arise in the third and fourth toe clefts where the toes are cramped together by tight shoes. A white, thickened, macerated area is seen and is tender to touch.

Seborrheic warts
They are also called seborrheic keratoses or less politely, senile warts. It is true that they are much commoner in old age but they also develop in people as young as twenty years. However, multiple examples on the back or chest are rare in young people. Seborrheic warts are harmless skin growths which have a rough or warty surface and vary from black to light brown in color. Telling them apart from other, more serious, growths is usually simple but occasionally it proves more difficult and the wart has to be removed and examined under a microscope.

Treating obvious seborrheic warts is only necessary should they be itchy or unsightly. Various methods can be used including cryotherapy, curettage or excision (see pages 46-48).

Serious lumps

Skin cancers

Skin cancer is already a common disease but we are seeing it more and more. There may be several reasons for this but an important one is that more fair-skinned people are being exposed to sunlight, either on holiday or having emigrated to a hot country. The problem is so great in subtropical Australia that almost every adult has at least one skin cancer in their life. Much more will be said about the damaging effect of sunlight on skin in another chapter but it is such an important subject that there is no harm in mentioning it twice.

To have the best chance of a cure of any skin cancer, early diagnosis is needed. Skin doctors have a head start on many of their colleagues in the detection of cancer because the skin is visible to patient and doctor alike. It should therefore be possible to pick up most tumors at an early stage of their development. That is why people are recommended to see their doctor sooner rather than later if they are worried.

Basal cell carcinomas (rodent ulcers)

This is by far the commonest skin cancer, and as suggested by the name it is derived from the basal cell layer of the epidermis. Middle-aged and elderly people are most likely to have the tumor but occasionally it may be found in people as young as twenty years. Too much ultraviolet from sunlight over a number of years is a factor. However, these ulcers also develop in people from cold climates who have never sunbathed in their lives.

The face, ears and neck are particularly disposed to developing rodent ulcers. The first sign is often an innocuous-looking whitish, translucent, slightly pearly lump. It may be pink and have an obvious dilated blood vessel running over the surface.It usually enlarges slightly before almost completely disappearing. This may happen again with the lump more obvious in its growth phase. An ulcer may form in the center, with some oozing or bleeding, but this may also heal temporarily. In other words it never heals but things happen so slowly that it is

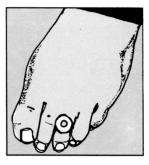

The treatment of corns should always start with removing the pressure factor. Regular use of corn plasters or paring will make them more comfortable but only a change of footwear can lead to a permanent solution. Corns on the soles can be helped by the use of spongy, soft inner soles or by the use of corn pads which help to take the weight off the tender center. However, advice from a physiotherapist or orthopedic surgeon may be needed to alter this pattern of weight bearing. Some people have a poor circulation to their feet e.g. diabétics or people with narrowing of the arteries: when these individuals have corns special attention is needed to prevent infection or ulceration.

often ignored for up to a year or two. By the time a doctor is consulted the rodent ulcer is often 0.5 to 1.0 centimeters (1/4 to 1/2 inch) in diameter. Fortunately these tumors never spread to distant parts of the body. They enlarge locally and eat away at the healthy surrounding tissues. They can damage the ear, eye, nose or any other structure and obviously should be treated before this happens. Most can easily be removed by a small operation under local anesthetic. Big tumors may require more difficult surgery, necessitating a stay in hospital and a general anesthetic. An alternative may be radiotherapy.

Squamous cell carcinoma

The cells responsible for these tumors are in the squamous cell layer of the epidermis. Like basal cell carcinomas, they develop on sun-damaged skin in most instances. However, they may be seen in individuals who have always avoided excessive sun and also on skin that is covered by clothes. Rarely, they also develop at the site of some previous skin damage - for example, previous scars from radiotherapy. Squamous tumors grow more quickly than rodent ulcers. The first sign is usually a pink or red lump. It tends to be irregular, hard and scaly on top and within a couple of months may be more than one centimeter in diameter. The center may break down to form an ulcer. Squamous cell carcinomas can spread to lymph glands or to other parts of the body, although fortunately they usually remain a local problem. This ability to spread means that rapid treatment is advisable.

If it is still small the tumor can readily be removed under local anesthetic. The site is important and it is easier to remove one from the neck, where there is often some loose skin, than from the nose or lip. Larger operations may require the use of a skin graft. An alternative treatment is radiotherapy but this is more often reserved for elderly patients.

Malignant melanoma

This form of skin cancer has a terrible reputation for several reasons. The number of people getting melanoma has nearly doubled in the last ten years. It can affect young people. It can spread to other parts of the body and show up years later. Lastly it may, in the early stages, be difficult to differentiate from normal moles and indeed the tumor may start in a previously harmless mole. This terrible reputation is, however, largely unjustified. Although less rare than it was, it is still not as common as basal cell or squamous cell carcinomas. Most malignant melanomas are diagnosed and removed in their early stages, in which case there is approximately a ninety-five per cent chance that they will cause no more trouble.

Malignant melanoma begins either as a new area of pigmentation or as a change in an existing mole. Any area of the body can be affected. Many existing moles change without there being a threat of melanoma, but certain appearances give grounds for suspicion and may warrant its removal for examination under a microscope. Worrying changes include much variation of the color, for example light brown, black and red brown; a jagged edge; recent increase in size. None of these changes guarantee that a mole has become malignant but they should prompt a visit to the doctor.

There has been much discussion in the media concerning melanoma. It has been part of a national campaign to make people more aware of the dangers of too much sunlight and to consult the doctor sooner rather than later if a mole seems to have changed. The obvious goal is to try and pick up most melanomas at a very early stage. It has a negative side because many people will start to worry about moles which are in fact harmless.

The effects of sunlight on the skin are discussed later but it is important to stress here that there is no doubt about the role of ultraviolet in causing malignant melanoma. Not everyone's tumor is due to sun but the more sun you get and the more often you burn the more likely you are to develop a melanoma. Just as heavy cigarette smoking seems hazardous today, so in years to come, sun worshipping may seem a stupid pastime.

When a melanoma has developed it should be treated by surgery. It is usual to remove some normal-looking skin around the tumor at the same time to be on the safe side.

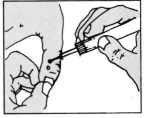

First, an electric current is used to heat a wire loop which is then placed on the skin.

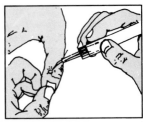

Secondly, a very high-frequency current is directed onto the skin from the tip of an 'electrode' and the current is converted into heat in the skin. These methods are useful to stop bleeding after scalpel or curette surgery; also small skin tags can be shriveled up and will fall off after a few days: local anesthetic may be required.

Treatment of skin lumps

Cryotherapy

The destruction of skin tumors by bringing the temperature well below freezing point is called cryosurgery. Liquid nitrogen is the most popular refrigerant (temperature in the flask -196°C). It is applied to the skin either on a cotton swab or as a spray through a nozzle from a flask. The use of liquid nitrogen for the treatment of warts is described elsewhere. Other uses are treating seborrheic warts, actinic keratoses (see under sun-induced skin changes) and occasionally small basal cell cancers.

Curette

This is best suited for tumors with clear margins and soft or firm consistency, like viral warts, seborrheic warts and actinic keratoses. Sometimes this technique is used to treat rodent ulcers but it is important to remove every fragment of tumor: the base is then cauterized to destroy any malignant cells that might remain.

Excision

The scalpel, with a sharp blade, is a time-honoured instrument for skin surgery. A local anesthetic is injected to make the skin numb. The simplest technique is called a biopsy: this is the removal of a piece of skin. The usual method is to make it slit-shaped, so that the gap can easily be closed with stitches. A small piece of skin may be removed as a curative procedure. When performing a biopsy due care must be given to the subsequent repair. If possible the scar should lie in an existing skin crease or wrinkle. It may be tempting to make a small round excision but the result of sewing up such a defect is often puckered at the ends. It is much easier to remove a tumor in areas of loose skin such as the armpit or the neck than in sites with no slack - for example the front of the shin. With increasing age the skin loses elasticity, as seen in the lined faces of the elderly, and surgery becomes easier.

When insufficient skin is available to remove a tumor and stitch the edges directly the services of a general surgeon or plastic surgeon may be required. The methods they use are of two types - flaps and grafts. Flaps are a clever way of using nearby loose skin to fill the defect. An example would be if a tumor the size of a penny piece was removed from the bridge of the nose. To fill the gap a similar-sized incision is made between the eyebrows but leaving the skin attached by a narrow stalk to maintain its blood supply. This piece of skin can be swung down to the bridge of the nose and stitched into place. There is now, of course, a defect between the eyebrows but this can be stitched together easily because the skin is much looser. Skin grafting is the transfer of skin from one body area to another. A graft may be the full thickness of the skin or only part of it, depending on the requirements. The donor and recipient skin must be matched for color, thickness and hairiness.

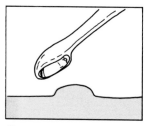

Curette
Shaped like a very small spoon with sharp edges, the curette is used to scoop out skin tumors: local anesthetic is injected first.

Lasers
Lasers produce very high-intensity energy either in the visible range - i.e. light - or the invisible range - e.g. infra-red. Increasing uses are being found for lasers in medicine. The energy from the laser is converted into heat that is used in much the same way as a scalpel. The main advantage is that blood vessels are sealed instantly so there is little bleeding. This is particularly useful in areas with a generous blood supply e.g. the tongue.

Radiotherapy
This is the treatment of tumors with various types of radiation, most commonly ionizing radiation, for example X-rays, beta rays or gamma rays. Both basal and squamous cell cancers may be treated in this way and there are many instances where it is the best form of treatment. Several treatments are given over the course of a week or two. There is no discomfort at the time but the skin may become inflamed at a later date. Radiation tends to be reserved for older patients because the scars, which are cosmetically good to begin with, can deteriorate over fifteen to twenty years and become unattractive.

Infections and infestations

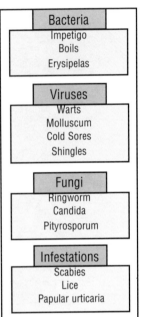

Bacteria
Impetigo
Boils
Erysipelas

Viruses
Warts
Molluscum
Cold Sores
Shingles

Fungi
Ringworm
Candida
Pityrosporum

Infestations
Scabies
Lice
Papular urticaria

This group of diseases is extremely common and no one goes through life without some infection of the skin at one time or another. In hot countries it is even more of a problem. An infection is caused by tiny organisms such as bacteria, viruses and fungi and can spread from one person to another. They are microscopic. An infestation, on the other hand, is caused by small creatures that can generally be seen with the naked eye.

Many of the microbes which cause infection are present in our everyday environment without causing trouble. Why then do they sometimes produce a disease? The answer is not simple but depends partly on the immunity or resistance of the individual. For instance, people with recurrent cold sores find they often have an attack during a cold, when they are very tired or 'run down', after an accident or under a lot of stress.

Avoidable conditions
It is commonly thought that many skin diseases are dirty, or in some way show that the sufferers do not look after themselves. This is far from the truth. Anyone can get boils, anyone can get athlete's foot, anyone can get scabies, although overcrowding makes scabies commoner and those with poor hygiene may be worst affected. To a large extent whether you get any of these infections depends on inherited factors such as your natural resistance, luck and how sensible other people are. For instance, someone with an active cold sore should not kiss people; those with athlete's foot or other forms of ringworm should not lend their towels.

Bacteria
Impetigo
This may be due to bacteria called Staphylococcus or Streptococcus or to both of them. Compared to a hundred years ago we see very little of this disease, probably because of increased standards of hygiene and nutrition. Only certain strains of these microbes will produce the disease whereas other strains may live harmlessly on the skin. Some people harbor the disease-producing strain in

the nostrils and from there it can spread to infect a scratch or a bite or graze etc.

It used to be common in rugby players and was known as one type of scrumpox. Transfer to other players was frequent. Another situation is people with atopic eczema (see chapter on eczema, page 74-85), who have very itchy skin - these individuals scratch a lot and impetigo often develops as a secondary event.

Boils

Some types of Staphylococcus bacteria can invade the hair follicles. If the damage occurs near the surface, a small yellow pus spot develops and will clear by itself in a few days. This is most often seen at sites of friction, e.g. in men on the thighs where it may be brought on by the rubbing action of trousers, damaging the hair. Other sites are the neck and armpits. A boil, or furuncle, is a deeper infection of the follicle and initially will appear as a tender red lump. After a few days the boil will point and discharge pus. A carbuncle is a group of boils which discharge through several openings. It is very sore and the sufferer often has fever and feels unwell.

A small boil causes little trouble but is more comfortable when protected: when it is just about to point it can be pierced with a clean needle and the pus gently let out. Some people have recurrent boils and very often the Staphylococcus lives in their own nose or around the genitals and anus. It is therefore important to avoid picking or scratching these areas because it will transfer the Staphylococcus to other skin areas.

Your doctor may prescribe antibiotics for a nasty boil and a carbuncle will probably need to be opened more than is possible with a needle. He or she may advise nasal antibiotics and antiseptics in the bath to clear the Staphylococci from your skin.

It may be necessary to treat the family in the same way because the bacteria quickly spread from one person to another. The final point is that people with recurrent boils sometimes have a lowered resistance and this should be checked.

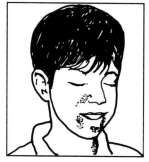

Impetigo
The spots start as thin-walled blisters which quickly burst, developing a golden crust, under which lies a red, weeping area. These crusty patches are most common on the face in children but, aided by scratching, may spread to other parts of the body and other people.

What to do
Avoid close contact with other people. This means children should be kept off school for a few days and in the household a separate flannel and towel must be used and boiled afterwards. The less it is scratched, the less it is spread around the body. Soak the crust off and apply an antibiotic ointment. See your doctor who can prescribe the ointment, e.g. Fucidin or Bactroban, and if the infection is extensive an antibiotic to be taken by mouth e.g. erythromycin. Impetigo should clear up quickly and there are rarely any further problems.

Erysipelas

The problem here is another type of Streptococcus bacterium which can get into the skin through tiny cracks. This may happen, for example, between the toes or under the ear lobes. No pus is formed by this microbe but the patient begins to feel ill and the affected skin becomes swollen and red and slowly spreads. This condition requires urgent antibiotic treatment - usually with penicillin (if the patient is not allergic to it).

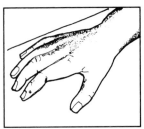

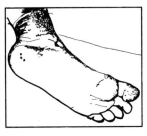

Warts are extremely common and are the subject of much folklore and myth. The word 'verruca' is the medical name for a wart, be it on the hand (top) or the foot (below).

Viruses

Viruses are even smaller than bacteria and fungi and they are not usually found on normal skin. Many viruses can cause a rash - e.g. measles and glandular fever - but these diseases are not dealt with here. This section describes some virus infections in which either the only signs or the commonest signs of the disease are on the skin.

Warts

It is now known that there are several strains of wart virus and each tends to produce its own type of wart. Some cause the ordinary wart on the hands, others painful warts on the feet; and still others warts on the face or genitals. Warts are caught from other people. This happens easily in children who have not had time to develop immunity to the virus but adults are more resistant. Even when the virus has gained access to the skin it may lie dormant for weeks or months before the wart itself appears.

Common warts are most frequently seen on the hands, fingers and knees. These may be one or many and a group may form into a large single wart. Because the virus spreads most easily into damaged skin it can take hold around the nail in nail biters: the appearance of multiple warty masses growing round many nails is typical of nail biters and pickers or people who manicure their fingers to excess.

Plane warts are almost flat and smooth and are colored like skin or slightly gray-brown. In some lights they may be difficult to see at all. Most often affected are the backs of the hands, face and shins and in some instances, large numbers may be found.

Filiform warts are slender, pointed warts often occurring singly and usually affecting the face, eyelids or nostrils.

Plantar warts, commonly known as verrucae, are found on the soles of the feet. There may be one or several. One type looks like multiple verrucae grouped together and is called a mosaic wart. Plantar warts are often picked up when the feet or floor is wet at swimming baths or showering after sport. Sometimes they are painful when walking. Another painful lump on the foot is a corn and this has a different treatment. Corns have a smooth surface and the normal pattern of skin markings (dermatoglyphics) is preserved. To distinguish the two a doctor or chiropodist may trim the surface with a scalpel and find that only warts have little black specks on the surface.

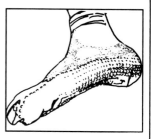

Rarely a wart may be removed under local anesthetic or injected with a drug which kills the virus. Fortunately this is rarely needed.

Genital warts are nearly always sexually transmitted and require a different line of treatment. This should include an examination of sex partners as well as looking for other sexually-acquired diseases. Various methods of treatment may be tried but it has to be regular and under supervision of a doctor.

Molluscum contagiosum

This is another common viral infection, sometimes referred to as 'water warts'. It is usually children who are affected and particularly those who have a tendency to eczema. The tiny spots are a whitish color and when looked at through a magnifying glass can be seen to have a small dimple in the center - like a doughnut. Multiple spots often appear and there may be some at different stages of development. Scratching fingers may spread the infection (see page 52).

Treating warts

The treatment of warts depends on the age of the individual and on the type of wart. Wart paints are the mainstay for common and plantar warts and when used properly go a are simple keratolytics, containing salicylic acid, which will gradually dissolve away the bulk of the wart. The wart is an overgrowth of keratin in response to the virus. Salactol, Duofilm and Verrugon all work in this way.

Warts: what to do
There is little you can do to avoid getting common warts. Nearly all children will catch them at school or from their friends but with plantar warts, steps can be taken. Lightweight rubber flip-flops worn in communal showers will prevent contact with the floor and a verruca sock (above) can be worn for swimming to reduce the risk of infecting other children. If you have scratches or cuts on the soles of your feet it is best not to go to the swimming pool.

It is important to realize that virtually every wart will eventually go away by itself: it may take a month or a year or two. When warts do go of their own accord they leave no scar or mark behind. From this point of view, any treatment which leads to scarring is therefore worse than doing nothing. It seems that 35 per cent of patients lose their warts within six months, 50 per cent within one year and 67 per cent within two years.

Molluscum: what to do
Molluscum: what to do
To prevent the virus spreading from one person to another within the family it is wise to prevent children from sharing the same baths, flannel or towel. Although the spots of molluscum go away by themselves, it may take many months. In adults it is possible to grasp the base of a molluscum with tweezers and squeeze out the contents, or - alternatively they can be frozen with liquid nitrogen. For children it is kinder to . soak the affected parts in a bath for ten minutes and then lightly scrub the top of the molluscum with a nail brush or pumice stone, while holding the surrounding skin taut.

Cold sores: what to do
Affected individuals should avoid kissing and sharing cups etc. Anyone who has had one episode of herpes is likely to get further ones. Prevention is difficult but one should try to avoid strong sunlight. Direct efforts at treating an attack as little more than a trivial nuisance. No treatment may be required or a simple antiseptic cream may be soothing. Some people find vinegar helpful.

Cold sores

Herpes simplex is the name given to an infection of the skin caused by a herpes virus. It is seen most often on the lips and face and called a cold sore. Almost any body site can be affected including the fingers and the eyes. Genital herpes is due to the same virus but will only be mentioned briefly here. With all herpes there is a so-called primary infection that may cause fever and general ill-health for a few days. After that the infection may reappear, at the same site, for the rest of life. The virus remains in the nerves supplying that part of the skin and can be reactivated by a number of factors, e.g. acute illness, sunlight, injury. The attack is often preceded by a few hours or a day of localized burning and tingling. The infection then reappears on the skin as small blisters on a red base in roughly the same place each time. They last for about four days, dry up and disappear without a blemish.

There is a specific treatment now available for *herpes simplex* that interferes with the replication of the virus. It cannot prevent future attacks but it can cut short the present one. Acyclovir (Zovirax is the trade name) is more effective as tablets than as a cream. It is often reserved for people who have severe attacks and must be taken at the first sign of itching or soreness to be effective. Genital herpes is acquired sexually and while it is active you should not have sex without a condom.

Shingles

Herpes zoster is the virus which causes both shingles and chickenpox. Having had chickenpox earlier in life the virus lives on close to the spinal cord in the nerves which supply the skin. At a later date, either when the resistance is low or for other unknown reasons, the virus spreads through the nerves and onto the skin supplied by that nerve. This explains why the rash is in a line, either down a limb or round the trunk. The attack is normally preceded for a day or two by burning or pain then the skin forms blisters on a red base that after a few days become pus-filled before turning into scabs. There may be some scarring. It is most worrying when the eye is involved.

Shingles is usually an unpleasant experience although some people have little or no pain. All ages may be affected but it is far commoner in the elderly. It does recur like cold sores. It may, however, give rise to a pain called post-herpetic neuralgia which appears within a week or two and may go on for months or years.

If the attack is recognized early the severity may be reduced if the doctor gives you acyclovir (Zovirax). However, if the blisters have been present for a day or two the medicine will be less effective.

Shingles: what to do
Many people find that simple painkillers are sufficient. Antiseptic creams may help to prevent secondary infection by bacteria.

Fungi

Several fungi can infect human skin, nails and hair. Those fungi which normally live in the soil or on animals tend to produce inflammation as well as scaling but those which are specifically human fungi give rise to little reaction on the skin. The term ringworm is used because many fungal infections produce a circular rash.

Ringworm

Ringworm on the foot is also called athlete's foot and it is the most widespread form of fungal infection. It is easily spread from one person to another and swimming baths and changing rooms are likely sources of infection. The usual changes are redness, scaling and maceration in the space between fourth and fifth toes, and it may be accompanied by small blisters. It may remain like this for years causing no discomfort, however, it may itch and spread to the other web spaces or other body sites.

Ringworm of the groin is particularly common in sportsmen and may be spread from one person to another by the sharing of a towel. Some fungi cause only slight redness and scaling whereas others may be associated with certain occupations in adults e.g. mining.

Ringworm of the nails
Ringworm of the nails is often seen with infection of the surrounding skin, but the most important causes of fungi

Ringworm: what to do
Ringworm of the foot is very common. Modern footwear is tight and leads to cramped toes with some friction. Infrequent washing and failure to dry between the toes favors the growth of fungus. The agents of ringworm are usually transmitted from person to person in skin scales shed on the floor. Anyone walking barefoot on the floor behind an infected person at swimming baths, shower rooms or at home is at risk. For ringworm of the body or scalp you should avoid contact with infected people or animals.
Treatment has become much more acceptable over the last twenty years. Colored antiseptic dyes and stinging ointments such as Whitfield's are rarely used. Your doctor can give you cosmetically acceptable creams such as Canesten, Daktarin or Exelderm, which quickly clear minor fungal infections. More extensive infections may require an oral preparation such as Griseofulvin which is taken for several weeks. Nail infections are more problematic. The tablets have to be taken until the nail has grown out - six to eight weeks for a thumbnail, eighteen months for a toenail. This, and the frequent tendency to reinfection, makes the treatment unsatisfactory.

invading the nail are trauma and poor circulation. The infection may enter at the free edge of the nail or to one side. Spread is progressively across the nail plate until most of it is involved. It may become thick, crumbly and discolored. Often only one nail is involved and it is usually a toenail.

Ringworm of the scalp and hair

A fungus called microsporum may cause bald, scaling patches on the scalp in children. It shows a green fluorescent color under ultraviolet light. Spread to other children at school is frequent so the child should be kept at home until treatment is well under way. Other fungi may cause inflamed, soggy areas with pus and hair loss.

Yeasts

The most important yeast is candida and infections caused by this microbe are commonly called 'thrush'. The yeast is constantly present but does not grow profusely unless there is a suitable warm and moist area of skin available. It favors the groin folds and armpits in overweight people, the skin under heavy breasts and the nappy area in babies. The result of candida overgrowth is red, glazed skin or sometimes a little scaling with eroded areas. These changes are more likely to appear in diabetics and those with a lowered resistance for other reasons.

What to do

Good hygiene helps to prevent thrush but it may be necessary to use anti-yeast creams such as Nystatin, Canesten or Daktarin. They are quickly effective but the yeast may return if the rolls of fat remain.

Infestations

Scabies

Scabies is an infection with a particular type of mite - *Sarcoptes scabie* - which is less than 1/20 inch long. The mite is passed from person to person by prolonged close contact. Holding hands for a time, sitting with an infested infant on your knee or sleeping with an infested person are the usual methods of transmission. The mites cannot survive for long in clothes or bedsheets.

Female mites burrow under the very top layer of skin (stratum corneum) where they lay their eggs. For four to six weeks there is no itching. But when it begins it soon dominates the picture and is particularly trying at night. Although the skin itches almost everywhere, with the exception of the head and neck, the mites in their burrows are found in only a few areas. These areas include the sides of the fingers and hands, the wrists, genitals, nipples and feet. A burrow is easily missed, being a gray-white line of no more than half an inch in length. The mite can be seen as a small dark dot at the end of the burrow.

Lice

Lice are insects and three types are partial to humans. They live in hairy areas and have legs which are especially adapted for grasping hairs. They feed on blood and inject their saliva. The puncture marks in the skin are the site of itching and sometimes bacterial infection is set off in this way. Each female louse lives about one month and lays up to ten eggs a day. These take a week to hatch and stick firmly, as small oval capsules, onto a hair shaft or strand of clothing material.

Head lice (*Pediculosus humanus*) are mostly found in children. Their eggs, or nits, are easily seen in scalp hair. There is often considerable itching and scratching and if a lot of infection develops the child may feel unwell.

Body lice are a subgroup of *Pediculosus humanus*. They are less common now and are seldom seen outside the unhygienic and socially deprived. Widespread itching and scratching may be followed by a pigmentation of the skin. The eggs are found mainly on the seams of clothing.

Pubic lice (*Phthirus pubis*) are common and tend to affect young adults. They are spread by sexual contact and by shared towels and clothes. Most of the eggs are found on the pubic hairs.

Scabies: what to do
Many people in a family or close contacts may be affected and the doctor will normally recommend that anyone at risk of infestation be treated. This is because it takes six weeks before you start itching in which time you could easily pass it on. Treatment works well. The lotion or cream (e.g. Quellada) has to be applied from the neck down. After twenty-four hours it should be washed off. After successful treatment it may take a few weeks before the itch finally disappears. People often think that the treatment has failed and re-treat themselves. This overuse can lead to an irritation of the skin with subsequent further itching.

What to do
In the case of head lice it should be remembered that spread from one person to another is by sharing hats, combs, brushes or close head to head contact. Body lice are transmitted by clothing or bedding. They need to be killed in the clothing by boiling, ironing the seams or dry cleaning. Apart from these measures it is necessary to apply an insecticide to the skin or hair. Gamma benzene hexachloride or malathion are effective for most lice infestations and can be bought without a prescription. It may be wise to repeat treatment weekly for a week or two in case further eggs hatch out. Other family members and classmates should be checked carefully for lice.

Papular urticaria
This is a skin problem affecting mainly children between the ages of two and seven but older children are occasionally seen with a rash. Red, firm pimples and blisters of various sizes lasting two to ten days are seen on the lower legs and sometimes the arms. They are in groups of ten. A sibling may have a similar problem. They result from insect bites to which the individuals have developed a marked sensitivity. The insects could be fleas, bed bugs, mosquitoes or house dust mites but may not be identified if they live on carpets and furnishings. Parents are often offended at the suggestion of insects in their house but there are few houses without some insects: the only change has been the onset of allergic reaction to the bites. To understand this it should be remembered that some people react strongly to mosquito bites while others do not. Fortunately, the strong skin reaction which produces papular urticaria settles in the end, but it may take months to do so.

Skin aging and sun

This is a topic close to everyone's heart. Many Western people are on the one hand increasingly conscious of their appearance and on the other hand doing irreversible damage to their skin by excessive sunbathing. Even sun-protected skin will age. Sunlight creates its own effect called photoaging, and the two processes together eventually lead to the typical changes of wrinkling, color variation and prominent blood vessels seen in old people who have spent much of their lives outdoors. We are now seeing this in younger individuals.In this chapter ultraviolet light and the changes it can effect will be discussed in detail, and then some of the theory behind skin aging and how to avoid it.

Ultraviolet light (UV)

Natural sunlight is made up of heat, visible light and ultraviolet light. The heat is essential for the warmth of our planet, the visible light for vision and photosynthesis in plants, but the ultraviolet is of less certain benefit. It does help to make vitamin D in the skin and insufficient can lead to rickets in children. Ultraviolet itself is divided into A (long-wave length), B (middle-wave length) and C (short-wave length which never gets through the atmosphere), but only the A and B are important here. They are abbreviated as UVA and UVB. The skin's response to UV is generally a protective one. Sunburn is a response to injury and suntan is a more effective protection because the melanin pigment absorbs UV. In tropical countries human skin has evolved to brown or black as a protective medium.

The dose of UV received by an individual depends on a large number of variables such as distance from the equator, time of year, time of day, cloud cover, reflective surfaces. You could burn badly in ten minutes in the highest UV conditions. Height above sea level is relevant because UVB is absorbed in the atmosphere: at high altitude there is a lot more UVB. Below sea level there is very little UVB, which explains why people can stay out for so long at resorts on the Dead Sea. They get plenty of UVA but it does not burn skin as effectively as UVB.

Sunlamps and sunbeds

All the problems which result from sunlight can appear as a result of excessive use of sunlamps or sunbeds. Naturally, the manufacturers of the equipment are going to point out the benefits of having an attractive suntan and feeling of well-being. They will mention that due care must be taken but they do not emphasize the long-term problems which include a speeding-up of skin aging. Artifical lights vary in the amount of infra-red, visible and ultraviolet that they give off. Most have some infra-red because it warms the skin and feels very nice. Most have some visible so that you know something is happening! The amount of UVB and UVA is variable but there will always be suitable instructions, which, if obeyed, will make sure you do not burn.

What follows in this chapter should give you sufficient knowledge of the effects of UV on the skin to persuade you that sunbeds or lamps at home are not a good thing. The only exception would be a specific recommendation, by a doctor, to buy one to treat a particular disease - e.g. psoriasis.

Skin aging and photoaging

As the percentage of over sixty-five-year olds in the population increases, the nature of aging and the diseases which it brings become more important. In addition, most older people have cosmetically annoying problems and many are the direct result of sun exposure over a lifetime. Normal aging leads to a loss of elasticity with fine wrinkles and a tendency to various harmless tumors and build up of certain cells - e.g. seborrheic warts. This occurs despite the fact that overall the cells are dividing more slowly. Also the number of sweat glands and blood vessels and the amount of fat is decreased.

Photoaging is important because it leads to color variation, wrinkles, prominent blood vessels and a variety of tumors, some of which are serious. Ultraviolet directly damages the cells of both epidermis and dermis. Some repair occurs, but over a period of time these cells show permanent damage and produce poor-quality collagen in the dermis and abnormal development in the epidermis.

Skin changes due to ultraviolet

Short-term

Sunburn

The main agent here is UVB. We are all familiar with the sight of a lobster-colored sunbather who has badly underestimated the sun's intensity or the amount of scattered radiation. It appears from thirty minutes to several hours after exposure and starts with redness and a burning sensation. In severe cases swelling and blistering appears, reaching a maximum on the second day, and in that situation some headache and fever are often present. It settles slowly and peeling is the last stage. There is no very effective treatment for sunburn, though wrapping the affected parts in water-soaked bandages is soothing.

Skin thickness

A few days after exposure the epidermis shows a slight increase in thickness and this may have a protective effect.

Pigmentation

The well-known suntan is the result of new melanin pigment in the epidermis which appears a few days after UVB exposure. It is an effective though not complete absorber of further UVB. People with the fairest skin may never tan but always burn. Most people redden a little before tanning but others never burn.

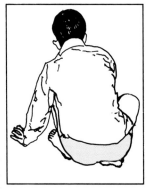

Long-term effects of UV

These can be divided into photoaging, potentially malignant and frankly malignant tumors. The changes result from a cumulative dose of UVB over many years. At present the worst affected are fair-skinned Britons who have been brought up in tropical or subtropical climates, e.g. Northern Australia or the southern states of the USA. Other groups include men who spent years in the desert in World War Two. The victims of the future are today's young men and women who roast themselves on sunny beaches every summer and who then try to maintain the tan by using sunbeds through the winter months.

Children and the sun
It is very important that parents should look after children's skin from an early age. Their skin is easily burnt and because they do not understand the need to be careful they would spend long hours in the sun unprotected. The methods are the same as for adults.

Cover children's backs and arms with long sleeved, cotton shirts to protect them from the sun.

Photoaging

Multiple small freckles appear together with rather larger and more pronounced flat brown spots often called liver spots. The skin shows unevenness in thickness and blood vessels become visible through the thinner areas: there is also unevenness of color with yellow or dirty yellow sheets appearing particularly on the temples, face and neck. It may become studded with blackheads and small white cysts. Not only do fine wrinkles appear but larger permanent furrows become a prominent feature around the eyes, mouth, forehead and neck.

Potentially malignant

Solar keratoses are sand-papery or barnacle-like areas of skin found mainly in fair-skinned people or after middle-age. The face, scalp (if bald), ears, neck and backs of the hands are the usual sites. Very early examples may only show a redness on the skin and late or well-developed ones can be large heaped-up tumors. They may be multiple or form a sheet over one to three square inches. There are two reasons for treating solar keratoses. First, they may be ugly, itchy or annoying because of their site, but secondly there is a small risk of transformation into a squamous cell cancer. This is really only a possibility in the larger ones with a red swollen base so treatment to all solar keratoses is not essential. Bowen's disease is a less common pre-malignant condition. It usually begins as a flat red scaly area which gradually enlarges with a well-defined edge. Any part of the body may be involved and more than one area may start simultaneously. The risk of change into a true skin cancer is very low.

Malignant tumors

Basal cell and squamous cell carcinoma and malignant melanoma are discussed in another chapter but they are all much commoner in people who have had much of sun exposure. The first two seem to be the result of a high cumulative dose over many years but the melanoma may stem more from skin which has been repeatedly burned. Melanoma is nearly twenty times commoner in whites than in blacks and it almost always occurs on sun-exposed skin.

What you can do

We are in a health-conscious age and one of the great advances has been a reduction in the number of adults who smoke. An equally simple remedy is available for those who wish to reduce drastically the risk of skin problems, including skin cancers. Strange though it may seem there are a lot of young people who are prepared to listen to advice because they are more worried about wrinkles than they are about skin cancers. Common-sense is one of the most important ingredients for success.

Awareness

Take note of the strength of the sun: i.e. how close you are to the equator, what is the time of day, what time of year is it, is there cloud cover, are there reflective surfaces such as sand or snow? Under the strongest UV conditions it may be sensible to spend only a few minutes unprotected in the sun. Noël Coward sensibly commented that only mad dogs and Englishmen go out in the midday sun.

What is safe?

There is no such thing as the right amount or wrong amount of sun. Everything is best in moderation and very few doctors will advise that you should not get any suntan at all. If you are on a one-week holiday there is probably not enough time to safely get much tan.

Skin type

Those with a very fair skin may not be able to tan at all, so there is little point in trying. If you do not tan you will build up no protection against the sun and will be burnt just as easily at the end of a holiday as at the start. People who never burn are luckier in this respect. UV will still age the skin and lead to other problems but to a lesser degree. It should not be forgotten that melanin only absorbs some of the UVB.

Shade

Visible light is reflected off various surfaces into the shade. It is not often appreciated that UV is reflected in a similar way and can burn your skin while in the shade.

Clothing

This must be the simplest way to protect the skin. A little UV can in fact penetrate some lightweight clothing but it remains a very useful way of blocking the worst effects. Hats protect much of the face and in bald people are most important. Sunglasses make life more comfortable but also protect the skin around the eyes. It is best to buy Polaroid lenses. Long-sleeved shirts and long trousers or skirts should be taken on hot holidays. After swimming in the sea it may be best to put on these garments until you next go in, especially at the start of a holiday.

Sunscreens

Competition between manufacturers has improved the quality and cosmetic acceptability of sunscreen products. No preparation is ideal: some are better at blocking UVB and others UV: some are relatively waterproof and will stay on during swimming or if you sweat a lot: some work by absorbing UV while others simply reflect it. The consumer must be guided by the information on the packet and the essence of this is the SPF (sun protection factor). A number from 1 to 20 approximates to the number of times longer that you can stay in the sun than you could do without this cream. In other words an SPF 8 cream, if properly applied, will allow someone who could normally stay out for fifteen minutes to stay out for two hours instead.

In America there are now SPF 60 creams but this reflects a tendency to over-react to the situation. In reality there seems little point in having a SPF of much greater than 15. It is certainly better to spend a few sunny hours indoors and the rest outdoors with SPF 15 than it is to lie in the sun all day covered in SPF 50! On the other hand, people living in hot climate (and this includes Southern England in good summers) should use a regular sunscreen.

Medical treatment of aging

There is no doubt that prevention is better than cure for all effects of UV on the skin. Premalignant and malignant problems can be dealt with by surgery, cryotherapy and radiotherapy (see pages 46-47). We are left with the aging skin and what can be done about that. In the last few years there has been a great stir revolving around a derivative of vitamin A called retinoic acid.Quite extensive experiments on animals have suggested that regular use of this compound as a cream can slow up the aging process of the skin or perhaps even reverse some of the earliest changes. Trials on humans have to an extent confirmed these ideas but it is difficult to get people to agree what are the physiological hallmarks of aging. Any hesitation and dialogue has been swept away, in the USA, by an overwhelming demand for the cream just in case it works. It is too early to say whether it does have protective properties for the skin but the sort of person who digs deep into their pocket to buy the cream is also likely to avoid excessive sun exposure.

Cosmetic surgeons come into their own when dealing with the ravages of time and sun. For them the market is enormous. There is no doubt that some operations are very effective at reducing wrinkles and furrows. The general term is a face lift and this operation tightens the skin; it does not make it young again. To get an idea of the likely result you should look into a mirror and gently pull the skin from the cheek towards your ear; and that from the forehead towards your hairline. Having established that such a maneuver makes things look better, the surgeon then makes incisions around the hairline and in front of the ears, frees the skin over the cheeks, gently tightens it, and removes redundant skin before sewing the area together again (see page 21).

Another technique is to inject an inert substance into wrinkles to make them flat with the rest of the skin. Collagen is the actual substance present in our own skin and the purified injection is made from cow's collagen. It is expensive and the effects only last a year or so before your body breaks down the collagen.

Hair and nails

Most of the time we take little notice of our hair and nails. During adolescence there may be times we would wish to have different colored or textured hair or curse that our nails break too easily, but after that we pretty well accept our lot. That is until some change occurs. When hair starts to be lost there is not only an immediate cosmetic problem but the scalp may be damaged by sunlight or low doorways. Equally, when finger nails fail to develop properly this problem is both cosmetic and functional: it may become impossible to pick up small objects.

Too little hair

Male-pattern baldness

This term is used because it is so much more marked in men than in women. The typical changes of receding hair and thinning on top are well known and often run in families: the process may even start before the age of thirty years. Women are much less severely affected and anyway tend to keep the front hair line. However, with increasing age many women notice some thinning on their scalp. The hair loss, in both sexes, is due to the effect of hormones but not an excess of them. The fault lies in the hair roots which become over-sensitive to existing hormone levels.

The first thing is to decide whether you want to try to hide or reverse the hair loss. Men are more used to the idea of balding and may accept it philosophically. It may be possible to alter the hair style, and shorter styles are often better. Dark-coloured dyes are counter-productive because the pale scalp shows through more clearly. Wigs or toupés find favor with some people.

A lotion containing minoxidil has been available for a couple of years. It is very expensive and not available through the National Health Service: it needs to be applied indefinitely. It may restore hair growth in some hair roots in a minority of balding people, but the benefits tend to be marginal.

Special forms of plastic surgery are also available in private clinics. Three techniques are used: the first is

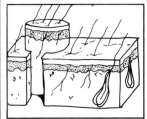

One of three surgical techniques is used. Small three to four millimeter circles are removed from hair-bearing areas at the back of the scalp: similar-sized circles are then removed from bald areas at the front and the hairy bits are inserted into the gaps. The procedure is rather like the transfer of small pot plants into a new flower bed.

illustrated in the left hand column. The second approach is for people with a prominent bald patch in the middle of the scalp. A bald area roughly 15 cms (6 ins) long and 5 cms (2 ins) wide can be cut out and the edges sewn together. Finally, there is a difficult technique in which a flap of hair bearing skin is moved forward to cover a bald area but without interrupting its blood supply.

Alopecia areata

This is the medical term for loss of hair in round patches. It may occasionally lead to a more widespread hair loss and, rarely, every hair may be lost from the body. No cause has been identified but the condition sometimes runs in families and may be associated with other diseases e.g. vitiligo (see Birthmarks and pigment). It usually starts in childhood or early adult life. Most of the bald patches regrow within a month or two but new ones may develop at the same time. Sadly, in a few people, there is little regrowth. Occasionally it is only pigmented hairs that fall out, leaving gray ones untouched, and when this happens people seem to go gray overnight.

It is never easy to be philosophical about a disease. This is certainly true when your hair is falling out. However, there is a very good chance that your hair will regrow normally even if there are a few further small bouts of hair loss along the way. Steroid creams and steroid injections, into the bald area, may speed things up. Ultraviolet light can also be useful. Otherwise, hair-pieces may be the only long-term solution.

Less common types of hair loss

Some hair styles may put a great pulling force on the hair root: these include some of the plaiting methods used by Africans. In Westerners the problem is usually seen in girls who twist their long hair around the fingers and pull on it. Scarring of the hair roots prevents any possible regrowth. It may occur in uncommon skin diseases such as lupus erythematosus, lichen planus, some infections and other rare diseases. Some of these may be treatable and should be diagnosed as early as possible in order to minimize the hair loss. Some serious diseases, such as cancer, may be treated with drugs which can also damage the hair roots. Complete baldness may develop within a few days but the hair starts to grow again quite quickly. After certain stresses to the body - e.g. pregnancy, illness, accident or operation - there can be a tendency for most scalp hairs to grow in unison. They are then shed at the same time, a couple of months later. The result is quite marked hair loss with a general thinning. Fortunately it is followed by regrowth.

Too much hair

Men have coarse hairs growing over a wider area than women. Hirsutism is the term for the growth of coarse hair on a woman, but in a male pattern. There is a wide variation of normal hairiness in women. For instance, some hairs on the upper lip, around the nipples, and on the lower legs are common enough to be normal. This is particularly true after the menopause. On the other hand, a heavy beard or growth on the chest is clearly abnormal but there is no easily identifiable point to distinguish between normal and abnormal. The problem is made more difficult by the considerable variation between different racial groups. Many Middle-Eastern and Mediterranean women have dark hair on the face and limbs. The first decision is whether to consult your doctor. If in doubt do so. The huge majority of excessively hairy women have no underlying disease. It is just part of their own development and may run in the family. Your doctor will be looking for some pointers which might indicate that there is an underlying problem. If the hirsutism has come on very suddenly, or your periods have stopped or you also appear to be infertile, your doctor might wish to do some blood tests. Otherwise, the decision whether to have treatment for excess hair is your own.

Local treatment
Shaving is a good treatment. Now that there are shavers marketed for women it has become a more acceptable

practice. Waxing is used for large areas, as on the legs, but must be repeated every couple of months. The hair is removed by the root and possibly a few may be permanently damaged in this way. It is quite painful and may produce infection around the follicles. Bleaching hairs makes them less obvious and is a method used by many people. The chemist may have a proprietary preparation but it is practicable to make your own one up at home: 50 ml hydrogen peroxide to 6 drops of ammonia solution, made into a paste with soap flakes. It should be applied to the skin for ten minutes before being washed off. Creams that loosen hair, thus enabling it to be pulled out, can irritate the skin and tend to be foul smelling. They are not widely used. Electrical methods are very popular but expensive. A fine needle is pushed down the side of the shaft and a tiny electric current passed which is converted into heat and destroys the root. Very few hairs regrow. The treatment is painful and most people can only tolerate a fifteen minute session. In that time between fifty and a hundred hairs can be treated. It is recommended that only a trained person uses this method (list of trained persons available from Institute of Electrolysis - see page 96).

Medical treatment
Very rarely the doctor will discover an underlying cause for the hirsutism. Treatment of that condition will then reduce the excess hair. When no underlying cause is found medical treatment is rarely recommended. Treatment, once started, would need to be given indefinitely and there tend to be side effects.

Nails
Finger nails take three to six months to grow and toe nails twelve to twenty-four months. Nail is made of keratin in much the same way as skin and hair. The visible part is quite inert and not much happens to it at that stage. The growing section lies mainly under the skin and the only part that can be seen is the half moon. Any disease which

affects the matrix, as the growing area is called, may produce a variety of changes.

Nails may alter as a result of an internal disease. Iron deficiency, for example, leads to flat nails and liver disease may produce white nails. Some medications produce discoloration. Other changes are seen in general skin diseases and some are mentioned in other chapters. Pits, like those on a thimble, sometimes occur in psoriasis and ridges and depressions may be a feature of eczema.

Brittle nails

There are many minor variations in nails which cannot be classified as diseases. In some people there is a tendency to splitting. The split may be wafer-like at the free edge of the nail or run longitudinally. Undoubtedly there is an inherited factor in some cases of fragile or brittle nails but it is usually an isolated problem. Whatever the cause it becomes worse after repeated wetting of the nails, so housewives are particularly prone to the problem. Some varnishes can damage the top layers of nail as can varnish removers. The best remedy is to wear rubber gloves over light cotton glove liners when in contact with water. Treatment with calcium, iron and vitamin E is often recommended but we do not see consistently good results.

Thick, hard toenails

Huge, thick, yellowy toenails may slowly appear in some elderly people. Occasionally a curly horn-like shape may be seen. These nails become impossible to cut and even chiropodists may have difficulty dealing with them. Older people may find they cannot reach their toes to cut them or poor eyesight makes it hazardous to try. Repeated damage to the nail over a lifetime and poor circulation are two factors that contribute to this condition.

Ingrowing toenails

This is usually only a problem of the big toenails but it may cause misery over a long period of time and seriously interfere with training in athletes. It is unusual before ten

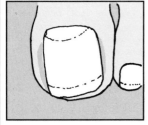

Ingrowing toenail
The nail digs into the skin on either side making it sore and often infected: sometimes there is an overgrowth of highly vascular tissue around the nail leaving an oozing surface. An acute episode of infection may require antibiotics.

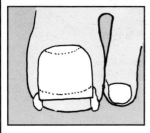

Other helpful measures include cutting the nail straight across and putting a small wad of cottonwool under the nail on either side. In the home it is best to avoid footwear when the problem is bad and generally to wear looser-fitting shoes.

and after twenty-five years of age and is never seen in races who walk barefoot. Ill-fitting shoes play a part and 'winkle pickers' were great offenders.

There are various ways of dealing more permanently with the problem. After numbing the toe with local anesthetic a strip of nail can be removed from each side, thus taking the pressure off the inflamed area. A further small operation to remove the matrix at each side will make sure that the nail never regrows.

Infection

Considering the amount of wear and tear which our fingers are exposed to, it is little wonder that the system fails at times. When people put their hands in and out of water many times a day the cuticle can be softened. In addition some people pick at their cuticles and damage them in that way. When an infection develops under the cuticle there is pain, swelling and pus seeps out: this is called paronychia. Antibiotics are the best solution in this acute stage. In people who do wet work the problem may become chronic and the skin surrounding the nail becomes permanently red, swollen and tender. Very often yeast organisms start to grow in the damaged skin and make the problem even more difficult to treat. The hands should be kept warm and dry; wearing cotton gloves under rubber gloves for work is helpful. Suitable creams to kill the yeasts may also be necessary.

Herpes virus, which normally affects the face giving cold sores, may also infect a finger around the nail: it is then called a herpatic whitlow. Swelling and pain, with little blisters, may last for a week or so.

Psoriasis

Types of psoriasis

The commonest form of this disease is plaque psoriasis and most sufferers have this type alone on and off for much of their lives. A few individuals will develop other varieties but this is usually a temporary occurrence which will then revert back to the plaque type.

Plaque (common psoriasis)

About one million people in Britain have psoriasis and the majority have the plaque form. The appearances are quite characteristic and there can be any number of patches, pink or pink-red, stuck onto the skin. They are clearly separated from the normal surrounding skin and come in almost every shape and size but tend not to have rounded edges. The surface is scaly and, on the legs, markedly so. The scale is silvery and is quite easily scraped off with a fingernail: however, new patches, those on the upper body and face, and those undergoing treatment may have little or no scale.

Skin over the point of the elbows and front of the knees is most often involved and both sides may be affected at once. The base of the spine and scalp are other common sites but, in fact, any part of the skin, hair and nails can be involved. Fortunately the majority of people have only a few sites affected at any one time.

Most psoriasis sufferers complain first about the appearance of their skin, but dry plaques, especially over joints, can split and be painful. Itching is not usually a problem, but for a few people can be very annoying. Scaling can be troublesome because it can lead to the shedding of dried skin flakes onto clothing or furniture. Some people with psoriasis are desperate to get rid of every last speck while others can quite happily get by with small plaques on their elbows and knees. The last group are luckier because psoriasis is so unpredictable it is impossible to say when it will go, if it will go and for how long it will be gone. It can come in short-lived attacks or grumble on for a year or more. Severe bouts may be short and mild bouts long-lived. You could say that there is no rhyme nor reason to explain the behavior

It is remarkable that a disease as common as psoriasis can be the subject of so much misunderstanding and ignorance. Almost two per cent of the population has psoriasis and yet for most people it is shrouded in mystery. Interest in the problem has increased markedly in the last five years partly because people are increasingly aware of their bodies and health but also because there is better treatment available. Research is beginning to unravel the mechanisms underlying the skin changes and hopefully will soon lead to a really effective and easy-to-use remedy.

An enormous amount of research into psoriasis has been carried out revealing many interesting findings. Some of the skin cells divide too quickly, new small blood vessels form in the skin, white blood cells are attracted to the site and the immune system is unusually active. But as yet we cannot fit all these changes together.

• Inheritance

Parents often ask what chance there is of psoriasis being handed on to their children. It is very difficult to answer because psoriasis is not handed down in a simple way like say, hemophilia. It is more like height, where tall parents tend to breed tall children but not always. We do know that if one parent has psoriasis then each child has roughly a twenty-five per cent risk of developing it at some time. If both parents are affected the risk is more like fifty per cent. We still do not know what is handed down to give the high chance of developing the rash. In identical twins, for example, it would seem natural that either one or both of them should get it but this is not always so. In other words, despite having the same genes, another factor comes into play.

• Infections

In the discussion of guttate psoriasis, an infection with streptococcus was mentioned as a trigger factor. Some people believe that other bacteria or viruses may act as a trigger for other forms of psoriasis. This would be one explanation of why only one of a set of identical twins develops the rash.

of psoriasis in different people. For this reason doctors are not prepared to predict the likely outcome of one person's disease. However, most people with psoriasis are likely to have problems off and on throughout life: there may be long periods of freedom but repeated spells of activity are almost inevitable.

Guttate psoriasis

This form of psoriasis occasionally appears a few weeks after a throat infection with a certain bacterium. In other people there may be no infection beforehand. It is not a common variety but the onset is dramatic. Hundreds of minute spots appear simultaneously and grow quickly. Usually without treatment it all subsides after six to eight weeks, but rarely it develops into more typical psoriasis.

Nail psoriasis

Psoriasis can affect the nail bed. Disease here leads to pits on the nail surface, separation of the nail from the nail bed at the end leading to air, dirt or infection getting in, or thickening of the nail to produce a yellowy color. Nail changes accompany other skin changes but occasionally they are the only signs of psoriasis. It may be difficult to distinguish psoriasis from other causes of nail change.

Flexural psoriasis

When patches of the disease appear in body creases such as the groins or armpits the normal scale is absent. A livid, sometimes shiny, red is usual and there is a greater chance of itching or soreness.

Pustular psoriasis

In a few situations groups of yellow-headed pustules develop. No bacteria are found in the fluid and the color is due to dead white blood cells. Perhaps the commonest situation is on the palms or soles and here, surprisingly, there may be no other evidence of psoriasis. This pattern is stubborn to treat. Alternatively pustules may develop on or around existing plaques and may be a response to over-enthusiastic treatment; or there may be widespread sheets of pustules and this is usually part of a nasty attack with fever and general ill-health. This form is very rare.

Living with psoriasis

Psoriasis can affect people in many ways at a physiological, emotional and physical level. Much depends on the way an individual copes with the problem.

Self-image is crucial to the way you project yourself. If a few small plaques of psoriasis seem to you to be a major problem, this will come across to other people. Nasty comments are frequently made in changing rooms, swimming pools or just in the street and only those who can brush it off as stupid ignorance will continue to feel any degree of self-confidence. However, the appearance of psoriasis on the face or hands may interfere with employment. A lot of skin scale may fall like a cloud of dust from involved scalps or legs onto the floor and be a social handicap. The feel of the skin may interfere when forming relationships with the opposite sex.

Most people treat their own psoriasis by using creams from the doctor. The longer you have psoriasis and the more interest you take in treatment, the more you can do for yourself. There are some important basic principles which are worth discussion and for these you do not need a doctor's help. The Psoriasis Association is an organization run by sufferers, and they have many experienced advisers (see page 96).

Holidays and sun

Many people find their psoriasis improves in the summer, particularly when on holiday. The beneficial side effects of ultraviolet light contribute to this improvement as do relaxation, exercise and decreased stress. Take all the holidays you are allowed.

General skin care

It may help to use a bath oil to get a film of oil onto your skin. Moisturizers help - E45, emulsifying ointment, aqueous creams are all good. Something stickier like Vaseline may be useful on plaques at times.

• Stress

The idea of skin diseases being caused by stress is an old one and usually a pretty unhelpful one. When someone develops psoriasis they often have to contend with comments such as, 'There must be something on your nerves'. Generally this is not true: stress is not the cause. In people with established psoriasis, stress can sometimes make it worse. Many diseases can be more troublesome at times of great stress or personal upheaval and psoriasis is no exception to this.

• Diet

There is nothing to indicate that any particular food or diet causes psoriasis.

• Things that make it worse

Some medications, prescribed by the doctor for other reasons, can make psoriasis worse. A group called beta blockers, used for blood pressure and angina, is one example and lithium, used for certain types of severe depression, is another. Scratching or injuring the skin may allow psoriasis to develop in the damaged areas. Sometimes when people are ill with another disease their psoriasis flares up but this is not invariable.

• **Ointments**
Stick to preparations that your doctor recommends rather than trying someone else's tube of cream. Most topicals come in various strengths - the weakest should be used first. Should skin develop a tolerance, a stronger one can be tried. If skin becomes red, sore or weepy stop treatment until redness settles then use the weaker strength again.

• **Tar preparations** *distilled from either coal and wood are very useful. They are black, messy substances but attempts to purify a clean fraction tend to lead to a loss of effect. On the whole, the smellier, stickier and blacker the preparations, the better the results! However, a compromise can be found in preparations such as Alphosyl, Carbodome and Clinitar. Pharmacists may also make up big tubs of dilute tar mixed with Vaseline. To protect clothes and bed linen old pyjamas can be worn or bandages wrapped over the ointment. Treatment is continued once or twice a day (according to your doctor's instructions) until the skin has returned to normal. Special mixtures are made for use on the scalp.They need to be washed out the following morning. A shower cap keeps the pillow clean.*

Scalp involvement is a nuisance and frequent hair-washing may be necessary - a short style makes this easier to cope with.

Clothing has to satisfy conflicting interests. Anything too thick and heavy will make you hot and may irritate the psoriasis. Most sufferers wear clothes that will cover the plaques, but you have to choose materials which do not become stained or greasy from contact with ointments.

Ultraviolet light or UV is divided into A, B, and C but only the first two are important here. UVA and UVB can have harmful effects (see page 57-62) but here we look at the beneficial ones. Many psoriasis sufferers notice an improvement in the sun and this effect can be reproduced by artificial UVB sources at home or in hospital. The effects are not readily explained. A low dose is given initially and gradually increased over a four to six week period. Slight redness may develop but is not essential for a good result.

UVA is less effective by itself but is usually combined with some pills called psoralens and the treatment is then named PUVA. The pills are taken two hours before exposure to UVA and this is repeated two or three times a week. Polaroid glasses must be worn for twenty-four hours after taking the pills to avoid damage to the eyes. This form of treatment is popular because it gets away from all the messy ointments. Caution is necessary whenever UV is used over a long period of time as it is known to age the skin and possibly increase the risk of developing a skin cancer later in life.

Admission to hospital

Most people with psoriasis never attend the hospital outpatient department and only very few ever require an admission to hospital. If, however, you have had psoriasis for a long time and simply cannot clear it at home despite intense effort and feel uncomfortable and miserable, then admission may be a welcome relief. The treatment is intensive, changes can be made on a day-to-day basis and the kind, knowledgeable approach of the nurses and doctors all help to speed up the clearance of the skin problems. It is possible to learn a lot about the treatment of psoriasis in a few weeks and this knowledge can stand you in good stead for years to come. Another reason for going into hospital is the very acute onset of sore psoriasis all over the body.

Tablets and injections

This is never the first line of treatment because psoriasis nearly always responds to ointments. Some people, however, have stubborn disease which never clears properly or it returns as soon as treatment is finished. Another group of people tend to get widespread pustular psoriasis. In these situations a pill or injection may be recommended and this form of treatment will normally be continued for months or years. The advantages are obvious, no time-consuming or messy treatment; no hospital admission; peace of mind that the disease is under control. The disadvantages are less obvious: repeated blood tests; several hospital attendances; some side effects.

Methotrexate is widely used. It can be given as a tablet or injection and is only taken once a week. Slight nausea may be a problem and a careful watch must be kept on blood tests to ensure that the bone marrow and liver are not damaged. Retinoids, in particular etretinate (Tigason) have been available for about eight years. Everyone will develop some dryness of the skin, lips and eyes, but other side effects are less common. The psoriasis gets much thinner and less noticeable but may still be visible as red patches. Blood tests must be checked for cholesterol and other fats and if they show a big rise, a change must be made in the diet or the dose of etretinate. Cyclosporin is the most recent addition to the list of useful drugs for psoriasis. The main side effect here is damage to the kidney. But, just as with methotrexate and etretinate, if the doctor keeps an eye open for side effects, there should be no long-term dangers from the use of this drug.

• **Dithranol,** a chemical made up in various cream and ointment bases, tended to be messy in the past. Recently the pharmaceutical industry has managed to make cleaner versions which are more popular, e.g. Dithrocream, but there are still problems. It can burn the skin and should always be started at a weak strength. Stains on clothes and linen cannot be washed out, and it stains the skin and hair although this fades quite quickly with time.

The usual starting strength is 0.1 or 0.25 per cent rubbed onto the psoriasis and not the surrounding skin. It may be washed off after thirty minutes or left overnight. This is repeated every day for a few days and then a stronger cream is substituted. If the skin gets sore, Vaseline can be applied for a few days.

• **Steroid preparations** are very popular with American doctors but less so in the UK. The advantages are that they are clean, stain-free and produce a rapid improvement. However, steroids can cause thinning of treated skin and psoriasis tends to reappear very quickly after treatment is stopped. They are particularly useful if the psoriasis is red and sore, or in a situation where rapid clearance is needed, e.g. just before getting married.

Eczema (dermatitis)

Although some people use the words eczema and dermatitis to mean different things, most skin doctors now use the words interchangeably and there is no suggestion that one implies an inherited factor rather than an environmental cause. Eczema comes from a Greek word meaning to 'boil out' and, as we shall see, this is a good description for one variety of the disease. Dermatitis means inflammation of the skin and this is also accurate.

Eczema is not a single disease but a group of irritating and sore conditions. In severe forms the skin may even weep and blister. There may be an inherited cause, an external trigger or a combination of events leading to the final picture. Eczema affects something like five million people in Britain in degrees from very mild to extremely severe, irregularly or persistently and in ages ranging from the newborn to old age. It is no wonder that a huge amount of money and time is spent on researching the causes and improving the care of sufferers. It is another example of a problem that may not kill people but causes a remarkable amount of suffering.

The most important types of eczema will be discussed in this chapter. Briefly they are atopic eczema (page 75-82): this has an inherited factor and produces a dry, itchy skin often reacting to wool, dust, cosmetics and changes in humidity or temperature; seborrheic eczema which is less itchy, may affect any age and usually involves the scalp (page 82); irritant contact which is a wear and tear problem often brought on by soaps, washing powders and certain industrial oils (page 82); allergic contact eczema which is a genuine allergy to an everyday item e.g. nickel, rubber or perfume (page 83-85) nappy rash (page 85).

Skin changes

Although there are several types of eczema they all produce comparable changes of inflammation in the skin. Some types are more likely to go on to the chronic stage and others may be itchier, and lead to more scratching, but under the microscope the initial changes are always similar.

Acute stage
The skin is red, hot, itchy, swollen and many small blisters may form. Most people experience a smarting pain. The surface is wet, particularly if the blisters burst, and this happens quite readily on all surfaces except the palms and soles - here the blisters have a thicker root and remain intact. The acute stage is usually brief and either settles or goes on to a more drawn-out subacute stage.

Subacute stage
Less discomfort is felt but iching may supervene. Swelling settles but dried fluids may produce a crust. Redness is prominent, showing that inflammation is still active. Bacteria on the skin surface multiply on the crusted surface and may penetrate through cracks, leading to infection. While it normally remains a localized problem the infection may spread and form a lymphangitis (this refers to a visible red line traveling up the limb to the lymph glands).

Chronic stage
If the cause of the eczema cannot be removed, or if treatment is not rapidly effective, the disease may enter a chronic stage. Vigorous and persistent scratching is directly responsible for the thickened, scaly areas which are the hallmark of this stage. The change is called lichenification and is a protective reaction against further damage.

We have seen that there are several types of eczema and that each can have acute and chronic stages. Although the eczemas and their treatment have much in common there remain important differences and it is best to discuss them one at a time. Atopic eczema is common and may be the most severe: many of the general principles of skin care are mentioned in this section.

Atopic eczema
Onset and inheritance
This type of eczema often starts in the first year of life,

though rarely before three months, but may begin at any age. It affects at least one baby in 50 and is usually mild.

Fortunately it clears up in most children by the age of four or five but it may linger on after the age of ten or rarely into adult life. There may be a long gap when it seems to have settled only to reappear. Doctors are very wary about predicting what will happen: for example, in the case of a baby with atopic eczema, there may be an eighty per cent chance of it clearing by the age of five. But that means one in five will not clear and the parents of that one will naturally be disappointed and lose faith in their practitioner. It is best to show a cautious optimism stressing the fact that a great deal can be done to improve eczema.

Atopic eczema often occurs in people with asthma and hay fever, or in their relatives. Not all family members will necessarily have the same problem. A parent may have hay fever only and each child may have eczema or asthma. The inheritance of these so-called atopic diseases is not simple. If one parent is affected there is a fifty per cent chance of each child developing an allergic disease. If both parents are affected the risk may be seventy-five per cent. It is remarkable, however, that sometimes only one member of a pair of identical twins may be allergic. This strongly suggests that in addition to inheritance, some other factor in the environment acts as a trigger.

What it looks and feels like

In a young baby the first sign may be an unhappy, restless child who rubs the face on the pillow but as soon as he or she can control the fingers, they are used for scratching. Red, scaly areas appear on the cheeks and behind the ears. Slightly older children often have crusted red areas on their ankles and wrists and by the age of three or four years, the folds of the elbows and skin behind the knees are usually involved. This latter pattern may persist into adult life. It is important to remember that most children are only mildly affected and may not be troubled by the slight dryness of their skin. The longer it goes on, the more likely it is that chronic changes will appear. The thickening and dryness start in the areas mentioned but can eventually spread more widely. Acute and chronic changes may exist together. All eczema sufferers go through good and bad stages and the reasons are not always obvious.

Itching is often severe and makes children very unhappy. The intense scratching and digging quickly leads to the appearance of raw scratch marks and bleeding areas. All this interferes with sleep and leads to chronic overtiredness and often failure to concentrate at school or work. Parents also get tired because they have to deal with an itchy, miserable and demanding child by day and a fretful, wakeful child at night.

Infection

The dry skin often has minute cracks through which bacteria can pass. Scratching makes this dry skin much worse. The usual bacterium causing trouble is *Staphylococcus aureus* and it may lead to yellow crusting areas or worse, to fever and pain.

Herpes is the virus that causes cold sores. Eczema sufferers often get more severe infection that spreads across the damaged skin and occasionally admission to hospital may be necessary. Two other viruses are those that cause warts and molluscum. They too may become more widespread in atopic individuals.

Living with atopic eczema

Affected people have to learn to live with their problem. It may be difficult to adjust but it makes life easier if you do. Teachers should be told of the problem, and so should other children's parents so that they can stop any teasing and help your child while he or she is away from home. Forming relationships may be awkward if your eczema is bad. It may be possible to hide badly affected areas by wearing suitable clothing.

Type of work is very important because some jobs can make eczema worse - e.g. hot, dry conditions - and it is important that the boss knows so that he or she can try and fit you in to a more suitable job. People often

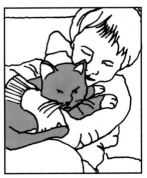

assume that the chlorine in swimming baths will aggravate eczema but in fact so long as you take a shower afterwards it should not be a problem. It may be a much greater problem later in life not to be able to swim.

What you can do about it

The more you know about the disease the easier it is to do what is best for your skin. Information is best obtained from your doctor, the National Eczema Society (see page 96), or a similar group. Reading articles in magazines often gives a distorted picture.

Pets are a problem. Cat and dog hairs may aggravate eczema and even rodents can affect some people. Bird feathers are also a potential problem so the choice of a pet is limited: a goldfish might be worth considering.

Clothes

Many synthetic materials and wool will irritate the skin so most eczema sufferers wear cotton whenever possible. It is smooth on the skin and feels cool, especially if loose fitting clothes are worn. You may be able to get all the clothes you require locally by using the Yellow pages and ringing around. Some specialist companies do a mail order sevice - e.g. Cotton On (see page 96).

Washing clothes is another source of trouble because the washing powders, bleaches and fabric conditioners may all irritate the skin. No product is ideal and some may suit most people but not everyone. It is very important to have a good rinsing facility so that all the detergent is washed out.

Housework and daily living

Many people with normal skin find that their skin dries out and cracks after a lot of dishwashing, clothes washing etc. Those with eczema have even greater trouble and should try to wear cotton gloves under rubber ones for wet work. Other chemicals may irritate the skin - e.g. polishes, aerosols, waxes - and care should be taken. Children may develop irritation from handling chalk, sand and other abrasive materials.

It is not a good idea to keep the house hot. Modern central heating and double glazing make it possible to have a very warm house but it usually makes itching worse.

Humidifiers are not recommended because they can increase the growth of moulds and house dust mites.

Dust
The dust mite lives in dust and there is reasonable evidence that some eczema sufferers are made worse by exposure to high levels of dust. This does not mean that everyone should obsessionally avoid dust but because it is difficult to predict who is affected some general measures are worthwhile. A good vacuum cleaner should be used regularly and in the bedroom damp dusting may be helpful. The heaviest load of dust mite is on bedding, furniture and carpets and in the bedroom it may be worth having a wooden or vinyl floor covering and no loose chair covers. Continental quilts and pillows should be filled with synthetic fibers.

Cosmetics
Care must be taken with all products that are used to make the skin look nicer, feel nicer or smell nicer. The skin of an atopic is more sensitive and may react badly even if it does not cause an allergy. However, I am not suggesting that atopics should not have the benefit and fun of using a wide range of cosmetics but care should be taken. It may be worth trying a small area on the arm first. When your skin is badly inflamed it is best to avoid cosmetics.

Leisure activities
Oils, paints, thinners and many other substances used for hobbies can damage the skin and should be avoided. Many sports are possible but for the worst affected contact sports such as rugby may prove very uncomfortable. Holidays are generally beneficial but be careful not to burn in the sun.

Forming relationships can be a problem. The relaxed enjoyment of meeting other people is overshadowed by itch, discomfort and self-consciousness about the appearance of your skin. There is no easy solution here but it is often helpful to talk to other people who have been in the same position and the National

Some general points are very important.
• *Finger nails must be kept short and smooth. Nails damage the skin during sleep as well as in the daytime.*
• *Do not borrow other people's treatments: get your own supply.*
• *Different body sites may require different strengths and consistency of cream or ointment.*
• *Follow the instructions from your doctor on how much and how often to use the treatment.*

Eczema Society will assist you. Sexual intercourse may be hampered by eczema affecting the genitals and your doctor should then be consulted.

Careers
Although most babies grow out of their atopic eczema there is often a tendency to have eczema on the hands later in life. For such people and especially those who continue to have extensive eczema, the advice is to avoid occupations causing much wear and tear to the hands. From this angle the worst jobs are as a mechanic, hairdresser, nurse or working with grease or oil.

Treatment
Most of the discussion in the last section was about excluding those things which make eczema worse. Here we will look at the useful things you can include. They are all designed to reduce itching and subsequent damage from scratching.

Moisturizers (emollients)
Dry skin is a common problem in eczema but is also found in people without eczema and is partly inherited, partly due to dry air, cold weather etc. Skin has natural moisturizing factors which maintains its elasticity. Moisturizers help both to retain the natural factors and to replace them. They are mixtures of water, waxes, fats and oils in varying proportions. Urea is a safe natural end-product from the metabolism of protein in the body which also has a strong water-binding capacity. It is used in some moisturizers.

Ointments are most helpful on very dry skin and work by preventing evaporation of water. They tend to leave the skin feeling a little greasy and to some people may only be acceptable overnight. Creams are nicer to use but the effect may be shortlived. Choice is definitely an individual matter and it may be necessary to try several before coming up with one that is satisfactory. Some examples of popular moisturizers are aqueous cream, emulsifying ointment, Boots E45, Diprobase, Hydromol,

Calmurid, Aquadrate, Unguentum Merck, Neutrogena hand cream and Alcoderm. They can be used as frequently as you wish. Children can learn very young to apply their own moisturizers and they often enjoy using those in a self-dispenser, e.g. Diprobase and Hydromol.

Tar preparations
They are not used much today except in tar bandages (see later) but they are effective in dry, thickened eczema. Ichthammol is also most popular in impregnated bandages but effective in relieving itch and soreness of inflamed skin.

Steroid preparations
They have a mixed reputation because when overused for long periods the strong ones can damage the skin. I explain to patients that alcohol also has side effects if used inappropriately but that most people can use it properly to their advantage. So it is with steroids. When simpler remedies have not worked they can be very useful. They reduce inflammation and itch.

Steroids come as creams or ointments and there are four strengths. Those known as mildly potent are suitable for the face, skin folds and occasionally longterm use. The moderately potent, potent and very potent ones should, by and large, be used for a shorter time and under a doctor's supervision. It is important not to get into the habit of using a steroid when a moisturizer would do the trick.

Bandaging
A bad bout of eczema can often be dramatically improved with bandages. They may be impregnated with tar, ichthamol or steroid. The immediate effect is cooling and they also prevent scratching. In the acute stage they will be changed every day but in the chronic phase they may be left on for a week.

Antihistamines
These drugs can be given as pills or syrup and reduce the

Bathing
Regular bathing is a good idea but it must not be an opportunity for the skin to dry out.
• The water should be warm but not hot.
• Stay in for about fifteen to twenty minutes.
• Avoid ordinary soap which is quite alkaline. Try e.g. Aveeno Bar (oilated), Neutrogena Dry Skin Formula, Sebamed.
• Add an emollient oil to the water. Examples that your doctor may recommend are Oilatum, Emulsiderm, Balneum.
• Pat the skin dry wth a soft towel.
• Showers are fine and bath oils can be rubbed into the skin.

Diet and atopic eczema
So much argument surrounds this subject that it is not easy to give uncontroversial advice. If there is a strong history of atopy in the family you should try to breastfeed your baby and wean later rather than earlier. Some foods like cow's milk or eggs do make eczema worse in a few babies but it is very uncommon and they tend to grow out of it by about four years old. If you think your child is affected discuss it with your doctor and do not substitute the food without discussion.

itching but do make you sleepy. This is acceptable overnight so long as the dose does not make you drowsy the next morning. They are safe in children.

Hair and scalp
Involvement with eczema is quite variable but usually a medicated shampoo is sufficient. Examples are T-Gel, Alphosyl, Polytar.

Seborrheic eczema
In babies seborrheic eczema may appear as cradle cap, a heaped mass of yellowy-brown scaling on the crown and forehead. Greasy scales may also appear behind the ears, face and other skin folds - e.g. nappy area, under the chin and the armpits. Even when it is quite extensive the baby feeds well and looks happy and mother can be reassured that it will settle within a few weeks. The cradle cap can be softened with olive oil and will come off in a few days. Other areas will respond well to a mildly potent steroid like hydrocortisone.

Adolescents and adults are usually affected on the scalp, central face, central chest and back. Dandruff is one form and minor degrees of scaling in the eyebrows and around the nose are common. There is often a greasy look to the skin. It tends to come and go and although, rarely, it is somewhat resistant to treatment, hydrocortisone creams are usually effective. Yeast organisms are known to grow readily on the skin and aiming treatment at them is often valuable - e.g. Daktacort, Canesten HC.

Irritant contact eczema
It is impossible to separate the different forms of eczema completely and atopics are more likely to develop the contact irritant type. In the general population some people are more liable to develop the irritant variety but it can develop in anyone if the stimulus is strong enough. The eczema appears when irritant substances inflame the skin. By far the commonest situation is when detergents,

soaps or other alkalis start to remove the normal fats and natural moisturizing substances from the skin. When this happens dry, red skin is seen on the backs of the hands and chapping appears with cracks. The fingertips are frequently involved and normal daily activities can further damage the skin. It is often called wear and tear eczema. An acute form produces small blisters on the hands and is known as pompholyx.

At home and at work
It is very common and may affect five per cent of the adult population. The skin trouble starts at the point where the irritant is at its highest concentration and this is nearly always on the hands. At home there is a large number of soaps, detergents etc. which can remove the fatty layer. Young mothers are at risk if they start to wash nappies by hand, on top of other domestic washing and cleaning. Indeed anyone who washes dishes regularly may develop dry hands with small cracks.

At work many people have their hands in and out of water (cleaners are an obvious example but hairdressers and nurses also have problems). Cement may affect men who work in the building trade, and oils can often be blamed in car mechanics and those in engineering.

What you can do about it
The most important aspect of care is avoidance. Clearly this is not always possible but every effort should be made to avoid the irritant substance. Protection is often feasible: at home rubber gloves can be worn for wet work (often with cotton inners), while at work a variety of specially fabricated gloves are available which are resistance to oils etc. Unfortunately many jobs require manual dexterity which may not be possible whilst wearing gloves.

The last aspect of care is treatment of the skin and the emphasis here is on the use of emollients. This has been described in detail in the last section. Steroids have a limited place in irritant dermatitis.

Allergic contact eczema

The problem here is an allergy to one or more substances that come into contact with the skin. There are important differences between allergic contact eczema and irritant eczema. In irritant eczema almost everyone would eventually develop a rash if they had to wash their hands twenty times a day in a strong detergent. On the other hand allergic eczema only appears in a small minority, however often they are exposed to it.

Many substances, known as allergens, can produce allergic eczema but the commonest are nickel (found in jewelry, watch straps, jean studs), rubber chemicals (gloves, clothes, shoes), colophony (sticking plaster), Balsam of Peru (perfume), paraphenylenediamine (hair dyes), wool alcohols (lanolin, cosmetics). The first signs of trouble often appear a week or so after contact but even if contact is regular it may take years before the body is sensitized and a rash appears. The rash begins at the site of contact but may then spread to other areas. Typical changes are those of itching and red scaly areas but blisters and weeping may occur in the acute stage.

Special problems

It is not always easy to know whether you have irritant or allergic contact eczema, especially if it is on your hands. Identifying the allergen is not always easy but trying to remember exactly when and where the rash first started can be very helpful. Even if you know the allergen there may be problems avoiding it because some chemicals are found in a huge range of everyday products. For example, you may develop eczema from epoxy resins found in some glues but then find that you react to other epoxy resins in electrical equipment, paints, fillers and resin films on plastic gloves and adhesive tapes.

What you can do about it

Quite often there is an obvious cause and an equally obvious solution. If you have just bought a new hair shampoo and two days after using it your forehead, eyelids and neck are all red and sore the answer is not to use the shampoo again. Likewise if a new deodorant leads to sore, itchy armpits you will be in no doubt about the cause. However, you may try another and find the same effect and then you do not know which ingredient is to blame. Alternatively there may be no obvious culprit for your eczema.

In these situations it is best to see your doctor who may suggest you see a specialist. In skin clinics quite a lot of detective work has to be done and is much aided by the use of the patch test. A series of the commonest culprits are put onto your back in a weak mixture with Vaseline and left under a dressing for forty-eight hours. If at that time a red, raised area of skin has developed under any of the test areas it is called a positive patch test and there is a good chance that the cause of your eczema has been discovered. If, for instance, you have hand eczema and your patch test to rubber chemicals was red and raised you may well be allergic to rubber gloves. The tests are not a hundred per cent accurate but they are very helpful. Having discovered a contact allergy there may need to be some adjustment to your activities, lifestyle or even work pattern. If it is something that you are handling at work there may need to be a move to another part of the factory or office. In addition your doctor will recommend emollients or steroid preparations to damp down the inflammation.

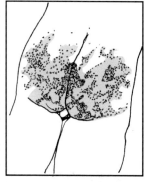

It is unusual for any baby to cruise through the first year of its life without developing a nappy rash. The changes may affect the creases alone or all of the skin in the nappy area, in some cases reaching the lower thighs. The color may be pink or red and the surface may be scaly, shiny or even covered with small ulcers.

Many factors tend to act together. A wet or soiled nappy and friction can damage skin if left in place for sufficiently long and then yeasts (candida) can grown on the damaged skin making matters worse. Seborrheic eczema and atopic eczema may also be the trigger factors.

Nappy rash

The baby's bottom should be kept clean by gentle wiping with cotton wool moistened with mild, unperfumed soap or cleansing cream. The skin should then be patted dry. The nappy should be changed frequently and as soon as possible if it is soiled. If towelling nappies are used they should be well washed and rinsed. A sticky ointment such as Zinc and Castor Oil can be applied to protect the damaged skin. Other treatments which may be recommended by your doctor or health visitor are antiseptic, anti-yeast preparations and hydrocortisone if it is very inflamed.

Alternative approaches

For alternative medicine, the skin is very much a reflection of our internal vitality, and skin disorders require a deeper assessment of ill-health or imbalance.

Acupuncture

Acupuncture regards ill-health as an imbalance in our distribution and use of energy, termed Chi. This energy circulates around the body in a pattern which the Chinese call meridians or channels. All our body functions are activated by this energy and are subject to two opposing but balancing forces termed Yin and Yang (for example, expansion and contraction, warmth and cold).

Herbal medicine

Although external applications are of value in soothing inflammation, reducing discomfort and combating infection, herbalists are concerned in establishing the links between skin symptoms and their deeper causes.

Homeopathy

The philosophy behind homeopathy is treating 'like with like', that is, using minute doses of remedies which, if given in large amounts to otherwise healthy people, would induce the same symptom picture.

Naturopathy

The key principles of naturopathy are correct nutrition and effective elimination of waste matter. As well as being a system in its own right, naturopathic ideas are an integral part of other therapies, especially herbal medicine.

Apart from changes in the diet itself, naturopaths increasingly use specific nutritional supplements to ensure adequate supply in the short term.

Osteopathy and chiropractic

Although these two systems of manipulative treatment have some differences, they are placed together here because they are likely to have a more limited role in the treatment of skin problems. However, in conditions such as psoriasis, there is often a strong link with arthritis.

Hormonal influence

Hormonal fluctuations can have quite a severe impact on the skin. Probably the most obvious example is that of acne where changing levels of sex hormones during adolescent years causes an over-activity of the sebaceous (oil-secreting) glands. If the glands and their associated hair follicles become blocked with sebum, then blackheads or pus-filled cysts appear. This can leave scarring.

Acne is usually a self-limiting condition (although this can mean several years; in rare cases it can be prolonged beyond the early twenties). The normal aim of treatment is to reduce the excess sebaceous gland activity and to significantly improve cleansing of the tissues.

In Chinese medicine, acne may well be described as wind and heat affecting the blood, and acupuncture treatment aims at cleansing or eliminating this imbalance. Interestingly, this idea of blood cleansing, although expressed in more conventional medical terms, is an important aspect of the approach of herbal medicine.

Herbalism can be particularly helpful for people with acne as there are a number of herbal remedies which effectively detoxify the tissues and improve the processes of metabolism; these are often termed 'blood purifiers'. Herbalists will also focus attention on nutrition, recognizing that diet alone does not cause the problem, but that dietary measures can be very useful, both for better nutrition and as part of a general cleansing and eliminative regime.

For the homeopath, dietary considerations and hygiene are also important, but the main emphasis of treatment will be to select a remedy for the constitutional imbalance, i.e. the individual's basic personality and responses to life and the skin condition.

In naturopathy, dietary change is the central platform for the cleansing of the inner environment and tissue nourishment. In addition, local measures such as compresses and friction rubs encourage better skin function.

Other areas of hormonal influence on skin vitality and appearance include changes as a result of pregnancy and also during and after the menopause. As far as pregnancy goes, any treatment program must be approached cautiously, with emphasis on dietary and other self-help measures for overall health and well-being, and perhaps external applications to help normalize the skin's activity.

During the menopause, hormonal changes bring about a speeding up of the normal aging process of the skin which commonly produces less oil. Acne rosacea, a condition with some damage to the skin, may be sparked off. The importance of the digestive system, especially the liver, is also crucial in creating this condition and needs to be looked at carefully.

Bacterial infections

Local or more generalized inflammation of the skin can occur from bacterial infection, such as a boil, or can be secondary to other conditions, as in acne. Boils occur when staphylococcal infection produces a large, inflamed, pus-containing swelling at a hair root. A multi-headed boil, or cluster of boils, is termed a carbuncle.

Despite the bacterial involvement in such conditions, routine use of antibiotics is not necessarily the best course of action, especially long-term antibiotic treatment for acne. The impact on gut flora, causing disturbances of bowel function, and the wider lowering of resistance to infection are warning signs that other options for treatment should be looked at.

All the alternative therapies discussed in this book would examine the deeper level of debility in a problem such as a boil. Diet is a fundamental factor, particularly excess consumption of sweet foods and alcohol. It should also be remembered that boils can arise as a result of more serious ill-health, for example, diabetes, so regular recurrences need to be investigated carefully. Touching or indeed lancing boils is not recommended, since the infection is easily spread.

As with acne, detoxification is the primary aim of treatment. Many similar eliminative approaches are used, as well as therapies to build up the immune system. This helps the body to cope better with the present infection and remove pus as well as increasing the resistance to future infections.

Impetigo is a highly infectious bacterial skin disease and sufferers need to be isolated. It generally affects school children. Blisters form on the face, often around the mouth and nose, and yellowish crusts appear on the skin's surface. Scrupulous attention to hygiene is vital in the treatment of impetigo, as is a thorough overhaul of diet, especially an increase in fresh fruit and vegetables. There will certainly be the need for local antiseptic applications, but once again there is a strong role for eliminative, digestive and constitutional treatment to increase vitality and health.

Our normal skin flora carries out a very effective job

of protection and warfare on potential pathogens, but the delicate balance can be disturbed. Unfortunately, antibiotics cannot differentiate between friendly and dangerous bacteria and a course of treatment may harm the skin's natural flora balance. Similarly, an excessive amount of toxins can build up on the surface of skin, most commonly from sweat imbalances. The most frequent symptom of this is body odour, as the bacteria struggle to break down the waste matter. Here too, the alternative therapies will look at the deeper disturbances causing such an imbalance, as well as paying attention to obvious matters such as hygiene and clothing.

Viral infections

Like bacterial infections, these can affect the vitality of the skin as a secondary factor, but they can also have direct effects, causing rashes and blisters as in the cases of chickenpox, measles and German measles in childhood and shingles in adults.

In all these conditions, alternative medicine does not aim at reducing the rashes because they represent the body's attempts to deal with the infection and remove the toxicity outwards. Treatment primarily focuses on

encouraging vitality, although management of aspects of the condition, such as fever, is important in therapy.

Chickenpox and shingles

Chickenpox and shingles are caused by the same virus, yet they are treated in quite different ways. Chickenpox is generally limited in duration lasting about a fortnight. As it is usually children who catch the infection, their underlying resistance and vigour is normally quite high. Thus, herbal treatment will look carefully at the need for fever management and gentle relaxation to calm the irritation and upset, as well as soothing preparation to put on the skin and ease the intense itching from the scabbing blisters which come out in crops over the scalp and trunk.

With shingles, the infection is focused on the nerve fibers, with painful blistering at the nerve endings, usually on one side of the face or trunk. Shingles strikes when a person has become generally weak and run down. Medical herbalists make full use of nervous restoratives to build up strength and vitality. Sufferers from this disorder often feel run down for some time afterwards unless they have some toning treatment.

Homeopaths are

interested in the total symptom picture for the individual in these viral conditions, for instance, whether the major problem is itching or heat and burning; what time of day or night the condition alters, for better or worse; how the patient reacts etc. By using a remedy which in large doses would give a matching symptom picture, the person's own defences are mobilized more efficiently.

In acupuncture treatment, it is the balance and flow of energy which is paramount and diseases such as shingles represent a deficiency of Chi, creating a weak condition. The dispersal of heat through the body is an important aspect of the treatment. For example, chickenpox is regarded as being caused by hot blood in Chinese medical terms.

Naturopathic treatments seek to manage any attendant fever in, say, measles or chickenpox, together with general gentle elimination and help through the convalescent stage, particularly important in the case of shingles.

Traditional medicine has a good deal to offer in the relief of fever and help throughout convalescence, and the naturopath will concentrate on diet and hydrotherapy.

Herpes simplex
Herpes simplex is related to

shingles and chickenpox. It causes small blisters around the mouth which burst forming yellowish crusts, often with cracks in the skin and bleeding. These in turn are prone to secondary infection. The same virus is also responsible for genital herpes which is easily transmitted through sexual intercourse.

Once again, a general lowering of resistance to infection is an important predisposing factor. Hormonal disturbances, stress and trauma, or local damage or infection of the skin also play their part. Therefore, treatment by alternative practitioners may range far beyond the local infection itself, correcting the underlying imbalances in the hormonal levels, boosting the immune system, or reducing the effects of stress.

Warts and verrucae

This is a very interesting example of the value of looking wider than the immediate skin problem. Despite being viral in origin and local in nature, they are strongly affected by other factors, especially stress and emotional upheaval.

The success of the old wart-charmers, still in evidence in rural areas or countries today, lay in the power of the mind over the body. By inducing a profound mental change, the warts were in some way rejected by the body's defences.

Certainly, warts can appear and disappear very rapidly with changes in health, and the immune-stimulating, cleansing and balancing approaches to the individual of the therapies outlined here can be very effective.

This does not, of course, mean that local treatment is of no value. There are a number of external applications, mostly herbal, which can be of tremendous use in clearing up warts. Medical herbalists will want, as will the other therapists, to assess vitality and treat the whole person alongside such applications.

Fungal infections

Fungus thrives when the conditions are warm and moist. A classic example of this is vaginal thrush, but these infections also occur when the body's defence capabilities are lowered. This can occur from a general lowering of health, from poor hygiene and over-restrictive clothing, and from some kinds of treatment such as antibiotics. It is therefore not surprising that alternative medicine encourages the immune system as a whole, as well as in some therapies having specifically anti-fungal local remedies.

Perhaps the most common fungal skin infection is athlete's foot, although ringworm, infections of the nail bed and similar conditions also occur. In all these, alternative practitioners concentrate on improving the body's natural immunity. This can be achieved by a variety of methods and in the first instance the naturopathic goal of enhanced elimination is of great value.

Hygiene is a key factor in athlete's foot and similar problems. A good circulation of air keeps the area dry and careful washing and drying is vital to prevent fungal growth. This is an area where the naturopath will be especially concerned and suggest an improving diet which feeds the immune system.

Herbal medicine uses these approaches too and will also use a range of herbal remedies locally and internally to enhance the body's anti-fungal defences. Homeopathy and acupuncture are chiefly concerned with the constitutional weaknesses that have led to susceptibility to fungal infection and will treat the individual accordingly for these longer-term imbalances.

Homeopaths do occasionally make use of local applications to support their internal treatment and of course in Chinese medicine herbal medicines and external preparations are often used alongside acupuncture.

Allergies

The whole subject of allergies is a complex one, with reactions ranging from an instant response to some external factor in the environment, to a long-term intolerance of a chemical or food. Essentially there is a hypersensitivity to one or several substances, and this can manifest itself on the skin as contact or allergic eczema, or perhaps as nettle rash.

A crucial element in the investigation and treatment by alternative practitioners of allergic eczema in particular is the role of any food allergies. Obviously, for the naturopath this will be central to treatment, but the other therapies also stress the need for this approach.

An investigation into the offending environmental constituents is also essential so that they are removed from the skin as far as possible. In many cases the irritant is clear from the area affected by the skin reaction - for example, watchstraps or rings made of certain metals. However, sometimes careful detection work is needed especially for less acute, generalized reactions. At the same time most of the therapies are concerned not only with finding and reducing exposure to the allergens, but also to altering the degree of hypersensitivity in the person as a whole.

Thus, herbal, homeopathic and acupuncture treatments will be directed at the individual internally as much as lessening the exposure to the environment or alleviating the external reactions with local applications. With nettle rash, for instance, there may be a relatively simple reaction to a single factor or a wider sensitivity, and often digestive disturbances are a vital element in the condition. By treating and correcting these, the problem can be resolved.

Eczema

The term eczema covers a number of inflammatory skin reactions to an irritant. As mentioned above, there are often several external irritants that can provoke eczema but there may well be internal factors also. There is also what is termed atopic eczema, a genetically inherited condition that usually starts to manifest in early infancy, although it may not begin till later in childhood. As this is such a complex condition, the insistence of all the natural therapies on treating the individual is clearly the obvious approach.

This condition is certainly made worse by stress, which provokes added itching and irritation from scratching the skin. The role of food allergies, most notably to dairy produce, is one that alternative therapies also pay great attention to in the overall assessment of this problem. Quite often the eczema is associated with asthma and /or hayfever and other reactions. This can occur in the one person or affect different members of the family.

As far as the skin inflammation itself is concerned, it tends to show up as either dry or weeping although it may progress between these two stages. In the former the main characteristics are a redness and thickening of the skin with a great deal of flaking and itching from the dryness. The latter stage is marked by an oozing discharge from the blisters and the skin appears more covered in the spotty rash than general inflammation.

In acupuncture, treatment is aimed at correcting the excess of damp and heat that is associated with eczema. This can often mean initially encouraging the skin to perspire more effectively - people who suffer from eczema often do not sweat easily, if at all. The movement of Chi, especially any stagnation of liver and/or lung energy, is of central concern and working on these subtle energetic disturbances produces a steady physical change.

For the naturopath, the person's digestive competence is a key factor and keen attention is paid to the prospect of food allergies complicating the condition. Diet and supplementation is geared towards ensuring effective nourishment of the skin tissues, and also to stimulate the liver and bowels to work more efficiently.

Herbalists are equally aware of the need for dietary overhaul, both to eliminate potential allergens or simply foods giving an excess of toxins and also to build up inner health. This is backed up by the prescribing of blood- cleansing herbal medicines which improve the assimilation of nutrients into the body and their transport to the cells. Once again, liver function is reviewed and encouraged and elimination by the bowels, bladder and lungs is enhanced to take some of the burden off the skin.

External herbal preparations are of value as well, both to soothe the irritation and reduce inflammation, and to begin to replace any cortisone creams which may have been used to suppress the problem. Indeed, long-term use of these cortisone creams is damaging to the skin, making it thinner.

The homeopathic approach to eczema is focused on the excessive dryness or irritability of the skin tissues, but even more so looking at the individual's reactions and general personality. For instance, much eczema is aggravated by stress and the dry heat of the skin may be a reflection of a heated temperament. By building up such a picture of a person, the homeopath will prescribe in highly diluted form, the remedy which gives a similar symptom picture in large doses.

Surprisingly perhaps there can be a role for the manipulative therapies of osteopathy or chiropractic in the treatment of some eczema sufferers. Restrictions of movement, for instance in the spine or rib cage, impede the blood and nerve supply to the organs and the skin.This could be corrected by manipulation and enhance skin function. Also, soft tissue manipulation and massage would encourage circulation and improve lymph drainage.

All in all the alternative approaches have a tremendous amount to offer people who have eczema and indeed are quite frequently sought by sufferers. There is no single magic cure for the problem partly because the condition is complex and varied, but there is great scope for finding the right horse for the course in the above treatments. Since eczema can come and go to some extent over time, caution should always be expressed about the condition having cleared up permanently but benefits are undoubtedly possible.

Psoriasis

Psoriasis is a particularly difficult and complicated skin condition. It is an example of an autoimmune disease when the body's defences start to attack its own tissues (other autoimmune diseases include rheumatoid arthritis and ulcerative collitis of the digestive tract). The reasons for this are not really known but it is important to thoroughly assess any history of chronic infections in the body - for example, persistent throat infections.

The ability of alternative medicine to make such links and to build up the depleted immune system which underlies such problems is a major factor in the improvements that natural therapies can bring about. The note of caution sounded with eczema applies even more to psoriasis - it is the individual analysis which is important.

Homeopathic diagnosis is directed at isolating the individual symptoms that will lead to the appropriate prescription. These are unlikely to vary in terms of the eruption itself, but in other aspects of health, reactions to illness etc. Since orthodox treatment may well have included steroid creams which mask any changes, it is usual for the homeopath to withdraw or reduce their use before giving the remedy. This is unless steroids have been used for a long time when a low potency may be prescribed during gradual weaning off the creams.

The medicinal herbalist would also be looking carefully at withdrawing steroid applications since prolonged heavy use can cause permanent skin damage. Herbal treatment will be started straight away, however, and will initially focus on the elimination of excess toxins, especially looking at liver and bowel function. An overhaul of diet, for instance reducing fatty, fried foods and alcohol, will complement this approach. This is accompanied by treatment of any chronic infection or weakness in the body's systems and by enhancing the person's ability to withstand stress. Since ultraviolet light is beneficial for the condition, herbal practitioners and colleagues in the other therapies will advocate plenty of sunshine - ultraviolet light is the basis for most intensive hospital treatment of psoriasis.

Traditional Chinese medicine relates the skin to the condition of the lung and the blood. The lung distributes defensive energy around the body, circulating underneath the skin, while the blood nourishes the skin. Consequently, any disorders of these areas would be tackled first by the acupuncturist, seeking to strengthen the Chi through the appropriate meridians or channels.

Naturopathy emphasizes that psoriasis is a whole-person disease and that a fragmentary, local approach will not get very far in the long-term treatment of the condition. Any predisposing disorders such as chronic tonsillitis, often noted in psoriasis sufferers, need attention and diet will be critical for the naturopathic approach. A short fast is often recommended to reduce the toxin load on the system, followed by dietary changes to improve nourishment and metabolism.

Some people with psoriasis develop a widespread arthritic condition, akin to rheumatoid arthritis. Since the latter is another manifestation of autoimmune disease this is not surprising and treatment will follow the above lines for most of the therapies. There may be scope for some manipulative adjustments, especially for any lesions affecting the nerves supplying the eliminative organs such as the kidneys, lungs and bowel.

Since conventional treatment of psoriasis is limited to suppressing or containing the symptoms, there is genuine scope for more positive approaches to the problem despite the complexity and stubborness of the disease, and those outlined above represent the major choices. The area of stress and psychological effects is one in which they and other therapies such as hypnotherapy or counseling can also offer much help, and this should go alongside the restoration of internal balance, digestive competence and so forth.

Skin cancer

Cancer is the general term to describe a condition where a group of cells start to multiply out of control and eventually invade otherwise healthy tissue. If this multiplication and spread continues unchecked and the cancer cells migrate throughout the whole body, then the condition is usually fatal. The key word here is 'unchecked', since on a daily basis some ten thousand cells become malignant - i.e. begin to multiply in this way - but they are dealt with by the body's defences.

Cancer has a number of differing types and forms, and is a great challenge to medicine of any kind. Often conventional treatment is of a drastic nature involving highly toxic chemotherapy, radiotherapy or surgery. It would be stupid to suggest that there are simple alternative cures, but there is a growing body of experience in gentler approaches to the problems. Often this is carried out by specialist centers such as the naturopathic cancer clinics on the Continent.

There are three areas where treatment can be directed: at the skin tumor or growth itself; by supporting and enhancing the body's defences, and by relieving the symptoms of the cancer by orthodox treatment. The first category is not a likely one for alternative therapies, especially since this will be where conventional treatments are focused, although there are a number of herbs that have some

potential here. It is in the other two categories that alternatives can play a large role.

The spread of malignant cells requires quite a major breakdown in our immune systems, and the rebuilding of these defences is a central plank of the natural approach to cancer. Of crucial importance is nutrition and all the cancer clinics have used this as a vital part of their treatment. This usually involves restricting many foods that overload our system with toxic residues and at the same time increasing consumption of foods like salads for maximum nourishment. Dietary supplements are likely to be important for the naturopathic regime.

Elimination is another key aspect in the natural approach and this is an area where herbal medicine can be very helpful. The medical herbalist would see increased elimination and immune enhancement as the prime ways to help the person's ability to fight back against cancer in general using tonic and supportive remedies initially to build up strength.

Chinese medicine too makes considerable use of herbal medicines to support immunity and control the cancer growth. This is used alongside acupuncture which

like the other alternative therapies is not only aimed at boosting the defences but also at relieving discomfort from the disease and from the side-effects of radiotherapy or chemotherapy.

Homeopathy is, as always, concerned with the strengthening of the basic constitution, giving the individual the vigor to attack and resist the cancer from within.

All these therapies are thus in their own way attempting to help the person rather than focus purely on the cancer itself, and they combine these treatments with naturopathic techniques of diet management. Alongside such methods is another vital component of the natural approach and that is using the power of the mind for self-healing and positive thought.

Most of the specialist clinics in particular employ counseling as a major tool for sorting out mental blocks and negative thoughts. Cancer is highly feared and its diagnosis can cause great upheavals in people's lives. One of the most fruitful areas of alternative work in recent years has been in positive visualization and imagery techniques which counselors, hypnotherapists and the like have developed. These not only help people to get themselves back into emotional balance and see the problem in perspective, but also enable them to do something themselves to tackle the malignancy.

All the above strategies are applicable in general to cancer, with individual variations, and skin cancers are no exception to this although often much more localized in their growth.

Alternative therapies are less concerned with the tumor itself and more with the person experiencing it, in contrast with conventional treatment which is aimed at attacking the cancer cells directly. As such, the best course of action may well be to pursue all the options that suit the particular individual.

Hair and scalp conditions

In alternative medicine, there is no special difference between conditions of the scalp and those of the skin in general, and the observations already made about treating the whole person and looking within for constitutional imbalances hold good here too. The state of the scalp will often reflect what is happening inside and in turn it will have an effect on the hair.

For specifically local skin problems like cradle cap in infants, or perhaps lice or scabies, external applications will have a significant part to play. The organisms responsible for the latter two conditions are highly resistant creatures which is why conventional treatment uses quite powerful chemicals. For alternative treatments to achieve results attention must be paid to the whole environment of the parasites with diet, hygiene and treatment aimed internally as well as any local (herbal) applications.

Once again, dandruff is something which responds to local measures, but also requires the whole-person approach of the alternative therapies. This condition is the result of a decomposition by bacteria of the sebum secreted by the hair follicles. It is often aggravated by the excessive use of medicated shampoos, or metal combs. The naturopath, acupuncturist, herbalist and homeopath will in their own ways look at cleansing and balancing the internal environment in order to correct elimination and disposal of wastes and supply the scalp with nutrients.

The condition of the hair, like that of the skin, can give important clues as to the general well-being of the individual. In times past the skin color, texture and appearance was of even greater consequence for diagnosis than today with all our laboratory tests. For Eastern systems of medicine like those in China or India this is still the case, but all the alternative therapies discussed will see skin and hair state as of importance. For instance, hormonal changes affect the oiliness of the hair, illness generally leads to some hair loss.

The most drastic change in the hair is of baldness. Although this is usually controlled by changing hormone levels in the body, particularly in men, it can be brought about by stress and each therapy has considerable resources to deal with this underlying problem, whether from a physical, energy-based or constitutional standpoint. Other illnesses causing excessive hair loss will also have options for their treatment.

There is no magical alternative for male-pattern baldness. The crucial importance of good circulation to the scalp is likely to be emphasized either with stimulating massage rubs and locally rubefacient (inducing redness) applications, or from within. Sustaining a person's vigour and energy may help, but of course we all follow our own path of hair loss and baldness itself does not indicate illness or poor health.

First aid

The skin is subject to constant stresses from the environment, with bruises, burns, stings, grazes and other wounds being commonplace. Alongside standard first aid treatments for these kinds of problem, or sometimes as alternatives to them, are a number of suggestions from other therapies, especially herbal medicine or homeopathy.

For example, mild bruising can be treated by cold compresses enhanced by the addition of essential oil of lavender. This can be backed up by comfrey ointment to speed up healing. Alternatively, a homeopathic dose of arnica may be taken to reduce the pain and swelling, with an arnica ointment to follow. An acupuncturist may use a moxa stick (a cigar-shaped stick made from compressed dried mugwort which is lit and made to smoulder) held close to the area to stimulate the blood and chi circulation, thus speeding up the dispersal of the bruising.

Minor burns, or areas of sunburn, can be treated by cooling the affected area for several minutes with cool and preferably running water. At this point alternative medicine can be very helpful. A few drops of essential oil of lavender will prevent blistering and speed up healing, or a choice of homeopathic ointments are available for mild burns.

Stings from bees or wasps can be a considerable nuisance during the summer months. Some people are allergic to the sting and any severe reaction requires urgent attention. Initial treatment is to remove the sting if still present and apply cold water or ice to the skin. For bee stings, using an alkaline preparation such as sodium bicarbonate solution will help, while wasp stings usually are soothed by a weak acid such as lemon juice or vinegar in water. Depending on the appearance of the area and other symptoms, the homeopath will prescribe a remedy for internal use. The medical herbalist may well recommend bathing the area with cool chamomile or marigold infusion, or diluted lavender oil.

Cuts, grazes and scratches are almost a part of everyday life, particularly for children, and demonstrate the capability of the skin to heal itself quite quickly. Conventional advice on cleaning the wound thoroughly would be echoed by all practitioners (diluted witch hazel can be useful for washing the area). There are a number of herbal or homeopathic ointments which will reduce inflammation and the chances of infection as well as speeding up healing.

For chilblains or in rare circumstances, frostbite, the circulation can be enhanced by infusions of warming herbs such as ginger or cinnamon. The latter condition, of course, needs professional attention quickly.

These examples serve to illustrate that alternative medicine has a good deal to offer in first aid and minor ailments affecting the skin. These generally fit alongside conventional treatments or advice, although on occasion they may be genuinely different options. Keeping the skin intact is more than a cosmetic exercise. For it to fulfil its many functions as effectively as possible it is essential that it is not impeded by infection, injury or other damage.

Other titles in the series

Your Active Body (ISBN 0 245-55070-4)
Your Sex Life (ISBN 0 245-55067-4)
Your Heart and Lungs (ISBN 0 245-55069-0)
Your Pregnancy and Childbirth (ISBN 0 245-55068-2)
Your Mind (ISBN 0 245-60008-6)
Your Diet (ISBN 0 245-60009-4)
Your Skin (ISBN 0 245-60010-8)
Your Child (ISBN 0 245-60011-6)

Available, Autumn 1990
Your Female Body (ISBN 0 245-60012-4)
Your Senses (ISBN 0 245-60013-2)
A-Z of Conditions and Drugs (ISBN 0 245-60014-0)

Useful organizations

The Psoriasis Association
7 Milton Street
Northampton
NN2 7JG

National Eczema Society
Tavistock House North
Tavistock Square
London
WC1H 9JR

The Institute of Electrolysis
6 Assheton Avenue
Audenshaw
Manchester
M34 5RS

Cotton On (for cotton clothes)
29 North Clifton Street
Lytham
Lancashire
FY8 5HW

The Disfigurement Guidance
Centre
Doreen Trust
52 Crossgate
Cupar
Fife
KY15 5HS

The Vitiligo Group
P.O. Box 99
London
SE21 8AW

Hairline International (for
people with hair problems)
Chantry Vellacott
Chartered Accountants
Post and Mail House
Colmore Circus
Birmingham
B4 6AT (enclose S.A.E.)

MGI PRIME HEALTH
Private Medical Insurance
Prime House
Barnett Wood Lane
Leatherhead
Surrey KT22 7BS
0372 386060